Dragon Sla
Lipstick

*Epic Tales of Women Who Have Slayed
Their Dragons and Rule Their Queendom*

*Melissa Mansfield-Anderson
Doree O'Neal Caroline Hammond Carla-Jayne
Hollingworth
Erin Moore Nosheen Khan Haley Gray
Melissa Carter Tequila Cousar*

Melissa Mansfield Anderson

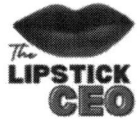

I would like to dedicate this work to the young version of myself and the young women that are finding their way through their dragon battles right now. When you are in the midst of the fiery breath of the scaly dragon and swinging a sword that seems far too heavy, know that you are capable, worthy, strong, and deserving of love and respect. You WILL be victorious in your battles—one sword swing at a time. You are not alone in this Queendom.

CONTENTS

Foreword

The Dragon Slayers Magical Queendom

As a Dragon Slayer myself, having slayed cancer and domestic violence abuse along with many other smaller Dragons along the way, I am so glad to know that although the dragons are big and mighty, we women are bigger, stronger and we wear a crown!

I would like to say a big thank you to Melissa Mansfield-Anderson for putting this fantastic collaboration book together and for including me in this important project of true stories of real-life female superheroes who rule their own destinies and queendoms, enduring many battle scars along the way but won proudly by all the authors. They teach us that we can rule each day with exceptional grace, resilience, and red lipstick too.

I can't think of a better read for women of all ages to experience right now in these turbulent and unsettling times. The dragon slayers in this book will uplift your spirits, giving you and your daughters hope that your future can be bright, as they each share their life-saving tools (weapons) of survival to help you accomplish whatever your goals are no matter what the size of the obstacles standing in front of you are or how hot the fire is breathing in your face from a dragon who thinks he can scare you.

I have said for decades that you can judge the size of the woman by the size of the obstacle it takes to stop her. Inside the chapters of this book, you will meet women across every walk of life, background, economic status, and regions of the world that all have this one very important thing in common, they chose to not let anything stop them. Going under, over, around, or through the biggest of dragons in order to be able to share their victorious stories with you here today.

With dragon slayers like each one of you who were brave enough to write your stories down in these pages, your legacy will live on and change lives for the better forever.

Living Happily Ever After…. or do they? You better turn this page now and find out.

Aurea McGarry

Dragon Slayer

Emmy Award-Winning TV Show Host & Podcaster

Cancer & Domestic Violence Sur-Thriver

www.AureaMcGarry.Com

Introduction

I am so excited to bring this book to you. The collection of women here within these pages is both diverse and powerful. We come from an array of backgrounds, races, and religions, yet all have our biggest strength in common ...we are Dragon Slaying women! We have each fought different battles, much like the ones you have fought or are still fighting. WARNING: This book is filled with triggers; suicide, domestic violence, sexual abuse, racism, and more, but each injustice is met with a powerful story of victory and a voice of compassion and help for you and the other women we have the opportunity to connect with.

As you read through all of the chapters or even just the ones that call to you, you will find our contact information at the end of each story. At one point or another, every single woman has needed the support of her female friends. Sometimes those friends are women you haven't met yet. It's us. We are those women. Grab a cup of your favorite beverage, snuggle into a cozy corner, slip into the bath or put your feet up somewhere in the sun and take some time getting inspired by the stories in this book that will remind you of YOUR dragon-slaying story you haven't told yet. With much love and respect, I tip my crown to you, you gorgeous creature of bravery. Always Melissa.

Welcome to the Queendom.

The Danger of Toxic Positivity

Smiles are dangerous, not for the receiver but for the giver. We hear it all the time. "Smile, it can't be that bad," "Smile, you'll be so much prettier." Between the Patriarchy and society, we are programmed as women that we have to just smile through it all. People want to do business with "happy" people. "Be the light in someone's day." But what about when you are the one that needs the light? THAT is when a smile can be so dangerous because that smile is hiding a deep darkness and a need for help that she is afraid or embarrassed to ask for.

By January 2020, I had built my digital company to exactly what I dreamed it should be. I was managing social media for restaurants, and I was doing contract work for an agency to design and build websites and create digital media for their larger contractors. I also had started teaching digital advertising as an accredited class to students at a local college.

Networking was actually FUN! Weekly meetings and lunches with other business owners and entrepreneurs kept me feeling alive and connected to the world of people around me. (I freaking LOVE eating food with others) It also gave me the opportunity to dress like I love, like I used to dress when we lived in Atlanta. I was at my me-iest me.

Valentine's Day 2020 was spent at one of my favorite restaurants, and one of the topics my husband and I discussed was the new rumblings about "the pandemic." I remember thinking that this would be just like all the other viruses that came before, "Mad Cow Disease" (I gave up beef for 2 years), H1N1, Bird Flu, etc. I had NO idea that this would be my last experience eating in a restaurant dining room for almost a year.

Three weeks later, I realized that there was a HUGE problem as the first of my restaurant clients cancelled their program. Slowly over the next month, all of my restaurant clients had to "pause" their social media management. A month later, they had to make the permanent decision to cancel their contracts. I saw what was happening to the food industry across the country and empathetically wished them well while I sat at my desk wondering how I would replace that income. I *smiled* and carried on.

Shortly after that, the agency that I was a vendor for had to make the hard decision of letting go of some of their contracted workers. I was on that list. Shit. The college? Well, we all know what happened with the education system. Still *smiling*, I carried on.

I had no idea what I was going to do. My experience over the last 23 plus years was in marketing and advertising, sales and design. I spent over 2 years working hard to build to where I was, and I was still growing. All of a sudden, I was at ZERO! I had a teenager, a toddler, and a husband that relied on me to contribute to our house. In disbelief, depression, and mental health fatigue, for the next three months, I dove into trying e-commerce retail.

I recognized that I was having a hard time, and I figured other women probably were, too, so I developed a small line of natural cosmetics with my best friend. I thought creating something I loved (makeup) would at least give me some passion. Plus, it gave me a chance to help other women feel good and express their feelings in a snarky way. It did. For 3 months, I created cosmetic formulas, packaging, branding, and labeling. To this day, I feel like that is what got me through mentally and emotionally while the world started to rip apart societally. I *smiled* as I tried to tell myself everything would be okay because it always "works out in the end."

We still own that little cosmetic company, Snarky Beauty, because of what it did for me and many other women at that time and even now. I kept a limited product line, and when I need a pick me up, I create a new flavor or shade. It's both excellent for my mental health and turns a part of my self-care into a small profit.

When August rolled around, I knew that I needed to be in a space where I could be back in the business-to-business world without so much overhead, translation, and I needed profit margin to pay bills. I invested in taking every class, course, and webinar that could teach me how to put my business online. I was so overwhelmed with all of the "new to me" technology that was required to run an online business smoothly. *Smiling* (and occasionally crying in the car when I was alone), I devoured it all piece by piece, and by the end of September, I had my new plan. I thought.

Like many other couples, after months of isolation and stress, my marriage was beginning to suffer under the weight of constant pressure of financial uncertainty, fear for the health of our family, my husband being an essential worker, and having to be in public all week and all of us having to stay home. Our joint personal account and my business accounts were constantly trying to save each other as I moved money around to make sure everything got paid AND we had food.

Many of our conversations turned into arguments, and during the day, it would continue through text. We had so much we were both dealing with. I now know that we were not alone in this struggle; any married person that had any issues prior to the pandemic saw how it seemed to exacerbate everything. I had started using the shower as well as my car as my safe places to fall apart and cry regularly.

On October 3rd, we had been going back and forth in text, and it started to get a little angrier and more emotional. I stood in the living room looking at how chaotic our house had become with 3 adult-sized humans and a toddler running around. We had all stopped putting effort into trying to keep anything organized, and depression hung over all of us, except the toddler who was happy to be toddlersaurus-rexing every day in her own little blissful and demanding world. I physically felt it. Like something had broken, a dam inside me that was holding back all of the hopelessness that had been silently building up over the past 6 months. The wall I had built of "everything works out in the end" became a cheap paper towel trying to mop up a river of anxiety and depression. I slipped over the line into a place I never thought I would be as a mother, wife, daughter, friend, as the "strong woman."

I handed my 2 year-old to my 18 year-old and sent them to the front of the house while I went to the farthest room in the back of the house. I sat on the side of the bathtub and called the Suicide Hotline. For 45 minutes, I cried and cried. Snotty disgusting sobbing about how I felt like I had failed. Failed my children, failed my husband, failed my friends, failed the women who looked to me for inspiration. I had failed myself.

As I explained how I felt about everything going on around and inside me, she listened with empathy and let me know that they were fielding hundreds of these calls a WEEK. I have always hated the saying "Misery Loves Company," but at that very moment, for once in months, I didn't feel alone.

When I got off the phone, there was no rainbow, unicorn, butterfly, or an amazing positive thought to greet me; what was there was a new knowing that I could, in fact, get through all of this. That I wasn't alone, and if I ever felt this way in the future, there was someone I could talk to without judgement. I just needed to find the root of how I got to that point. I spent the next few days going over the months since the pandemic started and holding them up to new eyes, and here is what I found.

My marriage, like many others, had its own issues we were working on but when the pandemic hit, our energy had become redirected to something even bigger, survival in a world that had record numbers of amazing human beings dying every single day. Without the energy to work on us and adding the extra fear of what was going on around us and the deep need to keep our family healthy and housed, the relationship we all wanted to be the strongest became the one that was hurting the most. It was isolation inside isolation. I wouldn't be able to fix that in days or maybe even months; that was a long-term project, but I had the capacity to start the process. Next, I realized that never being around other adults for someone as social as I am had truly been damaging to me; I just hadn't realized to what level. Lastly, *my passion was gone.* The things I was doing to feed my "make an impact" fire had been stripped away in this new world. Even on bad days in the past, if I was working on something I was passionate about, it helped me get through them. There was nothing in the place that that fire used to be.

See, back in 2019, I had written my first book, called *Learn to Love Your Bum: The 6 Steps to ATTACK the Mountain of Self Esteem and Plant the Flag of Empowerment in its Ass.* That book kicked off my live women's events about survivorship, strength, women building each other up, and they fueled me to slay dragons and kickass so that I could show other women what they were capable of. These events were my biggest passion projects and helped local women make connections and find healing. I needed to figure out how I could do that again but also turn it into a business. It took almost 10 months, but I did it.

I founded The Lipstick CEO in February, starting it with a podcast. As that evolved and my connections across the globe grew, I began to get to know women from many other countries. I saw that each country had its own form of patriarchal oppression, and THIS I wanted to help with. I created a coaching program to help female entrepreneurs, coaches and consultants become best-selling authors and build a coaching program of their own around their passion and genius. Empowering them to make money using their own superpowers. I took my Super Women's Summit online in a virtual event and put together this book. I found my passion and a way to wake up every morning knowing I am making an impact on women who will pay it forward and make even more of an impact. The bonus is now I am making a living doing a blend of what I know AND what I love.

As I put the finishing touches on this chapter this morning, I am looking at the toddlersaurus-rex watching Barney and trying to convince the dog she just wants to give her a kiss in a newly furnished and clean living room. My 19 year-old is shuffling around the kitchen foraging for breakfast, and my husband is safely working from home, newly promoted.

Things are not perfect. My office is a disaster right now, so is the kitchen. Laundry has piled up due to wrapping up this project. My marriage is still in need of soothing and effort, but the difference is that now we have taken the time to have hard conversations and are moving forward, giving each other the energy, space, and love to heal. I am personally in counseling to deal with the little bugger thoughts that are trying to hide in the baseboard of my mind, spirit, and body, and my oldest is also now in counseling to deal with 2 years of being unable to leave a house full of his sister and parents while navigating becoming an adult and yes, I cry about once a week to let it all out. I know I am one of those "sensitive and emotional" people. I'm finally okay with not being okay all the time.

Remember at the beginning when I said that a smile is dangerous? It can be...when it is attached to a mask. You don't need to keep smiling. Let the people who love you see how you are really doing. It's okay to need help. It's okay to feel all the feelings. It's not okay to stay there silently.

Shit is hard right now, my lovely dragon-slaying sister. Be kind to yourself. Be patient with yourself. Allow yourself to accept that some parts of your life may feel upside down, but you are still winning. You are here. You are reading a book filled with women who, though they don't know you, relate to you and care for you, exactly as you are. You are part of a Queendom of strong-ass women who still need a hug when times are tough and to hear that it will, in fact, get better again.

Melissa Mansfield-Anderson

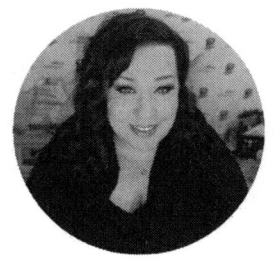

CEO of The Lipstick CEO

Story Mastery Coach

Independent Publisher

Melissa is a #1 International Amazon best selling author and national empowerment speaker. Melissa helps female coaches and consultants write their story in a best selling Battle Book© or in a collaboration book with other women Dragon Slayers. Her clients then work with her to build out powerful coaching programs and land their first clients. She is able to help her clients achieve success quickly, so that they can be making an impact with their passion and a profit with their genius, without months of overwhelm or overthinking.

Melissa is highly sought after for her experience in helping women tell their most powerful stories as well as making the messaging and technology portion of online business easy for her clients to understand and execute.

TheLipstickCEO.com

National Suicide Prevention Lifeline 800-273-8255

Crisis Text Line Text HOME to 741741 to connect to a Crisis Counselor

National Suicide Prevention Helpline UK 0800 689 5652

From Bullied To Badass

When I was asked to participate in writing a chapter in this book, the first word that came to my mind was bully. I knew there was something on my heart I had to share. The story I am about to tell is not one that I have told many people for fear of judgement. But in order to tell my story, I need to tell you the good that has come of being a victim of being bullied, but first, I need to share with you the darkness.

The word bullying has become a word that everyone can define. And in a world where cyberbullying has run rampant, teenagers especially seem to be falling victim. Stories of suicide appear on the news. But this is not new.

Bullying has always been around, maybe just not so mainstream.

The late 1980s is when my nightmare began. It was the summer before my seventh-grade year. The year before the summer, I had been my normal status quo. I got good grades, thought I had good friends, and I enjoyed most things girls my age enjoyed, such as MTV, shirts that fell off the shoulder, Scott Baio, and staying out until dark with my friends in the neighborhood until our parents called us inside.

I had the "typical" childhood summer, but I was nowhere near typical. Deep down, I felt lonely, not thin enough... pretty much just not enough. I was starving for attention and wanted love. To quote the old cliche song, *I was looking for love in all the wrong places.*

And it was this particular summer where I found it. He was a neighborhood boy that I had known for a couple of years. He had huge dimples and a huge floppy grin that could make me get weak in the knees. I was desperate to get his attention. But he rarely noticed me and often treated me like one of the boys when he did.

I tried everything to get his attention. I pretended to like the things he liked and would try to dress the way that I thought he would notice me. Looking back, it is quite silly how I fell all over myself, desperately trying to get him to notice me as girlfriend material instead of just the chubby neighbor down the street.

The point was futile. He had his own crush for a girl that rode our school bus. She was pretty, thin, and dressed in the latest, coolest fashion.

She was a year older than I was, and I admired her and hated her at the same time.

She seemed to have it together. She was like Madonna, and I was like Jan Brady in a Madonna costume. She was also the talk of the neighborhood as the boys were infatuated with her. And in hindsight, I guess I was as well.

How was it that she was so popular and had the boys swooning? I wanted to know the draw. I had to know. One afternoon, that 7th grade summer, this became a topic of discussion with my next door neighbor. He was tall and thin and not someone that I had an interest in other than friendship. Besides, he had an on-again-off-again relationship with one of my friends.

Sitting on the trampoline, I sought his counsel. I asked him what she had that I did not. I then went into a monologue, declaring my undying love for the boy with the dimples and floppy smile. I asked my tall, guy friend what I could possibly do to get dimples to look my way.

He stared at me with a cheshire grin on his face. "You know what you have to do, right? You will need to be like the girl on the bus. Everyone knows that she goes all the way. Would you be willing to do that?"

At first, I thought I was a little speechless. Sex in our family was not an open conversation. The most I had really known about sex was it was a sin, and I was not allowed to do "it" until I was married. So to ask if I was ready was not a question I was really ready to answer. But he had a plan.

He told me that he would work it out. He would talk to dimples if I was willing to be with him first. I honestly can say that I did not want to, but I never protested and said yes. After all, I didn't want dimples to think I was inexperienced, and I had to be as good as the girl on the bus was.

And so it happened. That day, in my neighbor's brother's bedroom, with the Brian Adams song, *Everything I Do,* playing in the background, I let him do what he wanted to do. It was awkward and emotionless. There was no tenderness, no love. I just laid there staring at the ceiling, wondering why I had said that I would do this. This was not the way that I wanted it to be.

When it was over, I left his house, feeling used and terrible. As soon as I got home, I took a hot shower. I was disgusted at myself. I could not get the image out of my head. I can still remember the smell in the room. It took me almost 30 years before I could listen to that song again

I tried to pull myself together, hoping the end result would be worth the damage I had done. But my neighbor was the tip of the iceberg. As we know, boys around 12 to 14 are willing to go to any lengths to have their first sexual encounter, especially when they hear from a friend that it was so easy with the girl next door. The next time was not the dimples but another boy in the neighborhood that tried to disguise himself as a boyfriend.

Looking back, I wonder how I could have been so naive. I truly believe that my hunger for love and attention was so intense that I was not willing to see the truth. This boy was shy and seemed caring. He had the prettiest, clear blue eyes. He asked me to be his girlfriend, and eagerly, I said yes.

We were not together very long, maybe a week, when he started putting the moves on me. I knew I had no other choice. I had convinced myself that the only thing that I had to give him was sex, and I owed him sex for taking an interest in me. If I didn't do it, I knew he would leave me.

Within a couple of weeks, if that, we were alone, and it happened. This time, the experience was "different." I thought that I had a caring, loving relationship, and it made the act a bit better. I still felt the guilt as it was over and chastised myself for being such a "bad girl." And to add insult to my injury, within a week of it happening, he broke up with me. I was devastated, used, and damaged.

By this time, I gave up on any self-respect or with what my gut was telling me not to do. This must be what guys want, right? And if they are not going to stay, then the next one has to be the one. And so, it finally happened with Dimples.

Funny how to this day, I can go into detail about those first two encounters, but I can barely remember what happened with Dimples. Maybe because by this point, I had shut down and started running on an autopilot that would carry me through the next 30 years. What I do remember was that I was hoping and praying he would see me the way that I needed him to see me. I was hoping he would look and treat me like the girl on the school bus. Alas, there was no fairytale ending.

What I hoped would bring us together as boyfriend and girlfriend ripped what was left of a friendship apart. At the age of thirteen, I felt used and washed up. I went into the bedroom with these guys with low self-esteem and left with self-hatred. I hated who I was and hated what I had done. I was ashamed.

But being the good southern girl, I swept it under the rug and tried to pretend nothing had happened. The rest of the summer, I hung out with the same boys, riding bikes and going back to our childhood games of hide and seek, stick ball, and jumping on trampolines. But I was not the same. And the following year was going to test my resolve and my strength. I just did not know it yet.

As the summer slowly drew to a close, I naively thought that my summer escapades would stay between me and the boys. What do you think teenage boys would do? I soon found out.

As I walked onto the bus on the first day of school, all seemed "normal." I sat with the two girlfriends I sat with the year before, near the middle of the bus. The boys from the neighborhood walked onto the bus and headed straight to the back of the bus. As the bus roared out of our neighborhood, I was relieved. Nothing had been said. Okay, good.

However, the whispers from the back of the bus became deafening. The hairs on my neck began to stand on end as the wave of the rumor made its way to my seat. I knew it was there before I heard it.

There was a roar of laughter as the chatter got louder. I heard my name as the three boys in the back were getting fired up telling the story of their summer. I was stunned and did not move a muscle. I could feel my friends beginning to stare at me. *"God, can this bus not get us to school any faster?"* I thought.

I could see the school ahead. I rushed to the front of the bus when we got to the bus parking and prayed for the doors to hurry and open. I had to get out. I could not breathe. The doors opened and I ran into the school. I hoped that what was said on the bus would stay on the bus.

But things only got worse from there. It took less than half a day for the whole school to know what I did that summer. As I walked into the lunchroom, I could feel the eyes burning holes into the back of my head. There were whispers and some that boldly said "slut" as I walked by. I wanted to die.

The rest of the school year proceeded this way. Some days were worse than others. The boys on the bus made up songs about me and sang them as loud as they could on the bus. Girls would talk behind my back in the classroom. Some girls would shove me down the hallway. And a few would ask me how it felt to be such a big slut.

I kept wondering how this happened and praying I could just go back in time and make a different decision. I was looking for help, someone that could understand me and offer counsel. So, when the girl that rode the bus that I idolized sat next to me on the bus, I was relieved.

I was relieved until she looked at me and asked me how I could do such a thing. I asked, "But haven't you?" Her response was, "NO WAY!" I felt duped and ashamed. I wanted to become invisible.

The rest of the school year, I spent my days trying to shrink from being seen. I would cry on the bus ride home and would run into my house as soon as we were home. I begged my mom to please not make me go to school and would beg for rides to school when she would not allow me to stay home.

My grades soon started to take a turn from straight A's to C's, D's, and an F. My teachers did not seem to notice, and I am not sure my family did as no one in the adult world said a word. I was alone and hurting. I believed that I had no one to talk to. The thought occurred that I would rather die than continue with my life this way.

The feeling of dying felt easy and got stronger as the torture at school and on the bus continued. Killing myself felt like the only way to end the pain. And on a random Tuesday, I took a shotgun from my stepfather's gun safe. I was ready to take my life.

As I stood there, thoughts of my parents swirled through my fuzzy head. I do not know if it was the image of them or the fear of actually pulling the trigger that made me stop what I was doing. But whatever it was, I was able to put the gun down and walk away. That day, I realized that whatever this was, I could get through it.

I would love to say that it got easier. Some days were, but most were the same. With each day, something happened that I do not think the bullies anticipated. Each day, I got a little stronger, and a lot more resolved that I did not have to listen to their bullshit.

And luckily for me, today's story is tomorrow's old news. And by the end of the year, I was old news, and the bullies moved on to harassing someone else. Things got easier; however, they did not totally go away.

Throughout my high school career, I would occasionally get called names. The rumor mill still floated around about me, and the jokes were still told. If someone got upset with me, they would cut to the quick and throw out an old "Doree is a Slut" joke and go about their merry way. The difference was not as many people thought it was funny.

And soon, high school ended, and college began. The pain was deep and left a lot of scars; I carried these scars with me for a very, very long time. Feelings of not being enough became a part of my belief system.

And that belief system provided the perfect environment for my alcoholism to flourish. I am not saying these experiences made me an alcoholic, but what I am saying is that it was a catalyst. You see, the things that the bullies said ran through my head for many years until I finally became what they said I was. And little by little, my self-esteem was destroyed, and who I thought I could be was decimated.

But there was hope. Getting sober, I began the work to heal and to forgive myself for the decisions that I had made in the name of love. I learned that we all do things to be accepted and loved. As my resolve grew stronger and my inner badass started to emerge, I realized the key truths.

First, bullies have their own demons to contend with. Bullies are insecure. Bullies are afraid, and bullies feel as if they are not enough. Second, a bully's defense mechanism is to tear other people down. Knowing this, the hate in me for the ones that had hurt me began to soften and turned into compassion.

It has taken years to heal. If I had been able to get past the pain and to be able to see the lies, I may have been able to heal faster. Seeing the bullies as the fearful people they are has helped me to recover from the trauma. They lie to others to cover their own truth. Their truth is that they feel they do not matter and they are not enough; the exact way they made me feel for quite some time.

But here I am now. I am no longer the person they were able to push around. And the joke is on them. They helped make me into the person I am today. I am now the person that helps others heal from trauma. Because of my experience, I had to dig deeper than I ever would have to find out who I am and what I am made of. My resolution is strong. My spirit is high. So thank you, bullies, for testing me. I passed!

Doree O'Neal

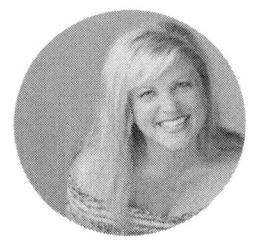 Transformation and Recovery Coach

Doree O'Neal is #1 Amazon Best Selling author, an inspirational speaker, and a transformation coach. She specializes in helping women that have recovered from addiction to find the lives they got sober for and women that have lost their way on the path to being a daring badass.

Her first book, Seriously? How I Went from a Hot Mess to a Daring Bad Ass, was her way of sharing her personal experiences with alcoholism and recovery, surviving an abusive relationship, and how she let go of self-destructive behaviors. Through her own healing process, she was also able to discover her joy and happiness. She holds two bachelor's degrees, two master's degrees and will be working toward her doctorate in Metaphysical Science.

She is a strong believer that we are on this earth to thrive, not just survive. She believes self-exploration is where the healing begins. Doree is a grateful, recovering, thriving woman that is ready to fulfill her life purpose of helping others.

TheRealDoreeO.com

https://www.stopbullying.gov/

https://www.cfchildren.org/resources/bullying-prevention-resources/

The Ever-Present Dragon

My dragon? Let me tell you about my dragon. To set the mood, my friends, we really have to create a vibe. It's as if life's twists and turns have brought you and I here to this moment in time. Maybe we are having coffee. Maybe we had reservations at a cool speakeasy and are currently using a code to get into the secret bar. Maybe we randomly met at a conference where I just completed my program, and with a tentative approach and slight voice, you ask, "Can I talk to you?"

Or most likely, you decided to buy "Dragon Slayers Wear Lipstick" (thank you, by the way!) and are coming to my chapter of 'The Ever Present Dragon.'

Regardless of where or how (and I'd still like to believe the first paragraph here can still happen), we need a mood.

I have to start with music. Music is ever-present in my life and the life of my family. I have to tell you, our best family meals include making a huge Mexican feast with my daughter's most perfect pico do gallo, and Spotify's "70's Road Trip Radio" is turned up on the WONDERBOOM blue truth in the living room.

So, our mood song has to be Carole King's "I Feel the Earth Move." Now, I do believe Ms. King wrote the song about falling in love. Not me. Not here in this chapter. In this chapter, her song reminds me of my past life- my "before." I escaped the man who was abusing me and my family. The violence and disease, which were in my life for almost eight years, created an ever-present dragon that rose from the depths of soul-hurt.

"I feel the earth move under my feet

I feel the sky tumblin' down, a-tumblin' down

I feel the earth move under my feet

I feel the sky tumblin' down, a-tumblin' down

I just a-lose control

Down to my very soul

I get hot and cold

All over, all over, all over, all over

I feel the earth move under my feet

I feel the sky tumblin' down, a-tumblin' down

I feel the earth move under my feet

I feel the sky tumblin' down, tumblin' down

Tumblin' down, tumblin' down

Tumblin' down

Tumblin' down"

Yes, dear friends, this song is playing in the background, and the smell in the air is a masculine mix of red wine and leather, but with a cumulative eight years tinge of a fire pit burning outside.

Or maybe it's not the fire pit, but the ever-present flames just under the perfect facade of a sleeping dragon. Reality for people navigating abuse means the dragon is ever-present, only hiding itself from the outside world and even the person with whom a home is shared.

My dragon is my own personal nemesis of domestic violence, created to taunt me, even as the years roll by and healing takes form. The dragon is still there.

I know my dragon well, and the dragon knows me. It has multiple different heads and twelve tentacles coming out from around its back and sides. It's kind of like an octopus/dragon that breathes fire. It can also fly. Swiftly, from one situation to the next, breathing fire wherever it looks. This dragon stays in my head but becomes alive in the world via my thoughts and actions.

I firmly believe every different component of my story is just another tentacle ready to whip around and take my feet out from under me. In the years it has taken me to chart a path toward healing, those tentacles rise in an ugly 45 degree arc, and BAM! a beautiful day turns to tears and fear, and I'm left crying in aisle three of the grocery store as I try and pick out a good bottle of whiskey.

I can have my feet on the ground, firm and steady, ready to banish the dragon to hell, when

BAM! another tentacle and another head came out of nowhere, striking the pain of remembering past wounds straight into the present and affecting my relationships with other people in the now.

I can try and pivot quickly, do one of those kick-cartwheel-spins across the floor like I'm a ninja in an action movie, when BAM! my world can grow dark and menacing, and I cancel all plans to stay home in bed overeating and drinking too much by myself.

I was powerless to control the dragon, just as I was powerless to control the actions of the man who claimed to love me, created a life with me, and blended a family with me, all the while issuing horrific abuse at home and living a secret double life at every opportunity he could create.

All the ugly heads of the one dragon I chose to slay could keep us together talking for an entire weekend. I mean, it would be cool to hang out with you because I'm thinking you're a survivor, too. Maybe not domestic violence, but maybe life's journey lifted you high in the air and figuratively bounced you back down on a grassy spot, only to repeat the process again and again. Regardless of your dragon, I'm sure we'd be friends. Dragon Slayers are the coolest damn people on the planet.

So for today's chat, I'm picking one head of the ugly dragon- the "Why Didn't They Just Leave" head.

Let's use my imagination here. Create the picture, in your brain, of me getting to slay this dragon. I'm leaning back on my left leg, striking a pose like I am getting ready to swing on a perfect pitch with a 3-2 count in softball, but I'm not holding a bat in my hand. Instead, I have a four foot long, beautifully crafted sword made from a winner of the Forged In Fire TV show! It even seems to be glowing gold-red when the sun hits the sword on this particularly beautiful day.

I decided to expose this dragon's head to its death when a filmmaker named Anastazja Gajkowska interviewed me for her documentary entitled "Expose- Express Your Truth," which should premiere in 2022. Anastazja asked me a question no one had ever asked me before, along this pathway of navigating domestic violence and the healing which comes "after."

Her question? "What attracted you to this man, who ultimately abused you?"

I laughed out loud because I haven't seen him in years, and the images I have of him now are of a shriveled up, meek troll-man with horrible nasty bad breath, who walks with a limp, can't seem to get it up (his back, but other body parts, too) and never looks someone in the eye. When I see old pictures of him in my mountains of evidence, it's what I see now, too. Even in his suit and tie. Troll.

But Anastazja prodded further, "No, Caroline. What attracted you to him in the beginning?"

Wow! Ok. Well, let's head back there (I have to admit the question felt like another dragon tail sucker punch from the left side, where my peripheral vision isn't good.)

I thought he was handsome, not in a Ryan Reynolds kind of way, but rather because of his intelligence. I don't think any of my friends looked at him and thought, "Oh my goddddddd! He is so handsome!" but he was super smart, and I liked the way he put together a sentence.

I'd known him forever, and we reconnected after both of our divorces, so the history certainly helped define the relationship.

Really, though, it was how he made me feel.

The relationship began as a fairy tale—all love, laughter, fun, and adventure. We traveled. We held hands. We danced naked. And every night, even if we were fighting, we fell asleep all tangled up with each other in bed.

He once announced our love was so huge and massive, and we needed to create a new word for this incredible love, or maybe a code word where only the two of us secretly knew the intimately incredible love we had when the word was said.

This person who would eventually issue horrific abuse against me also began as a completely vulnerable and open book about all of his life's challenges. He had never been understood by his family. He had never really been in love with his first wife, and no person on this earth had ever given the kind of love I provided. I was his savior and the only woman who could help him rebuild his life from all the crazy he had lived before me. He needed me to be his because I was his soul mate, and he finally found me.

He would share intimate details of his family life with the ever-present, "I've never told anyone this before, but I love you so much and feel safe with you." Details which made him cry and seem so wounded and vulnerable in my arms.

"I love you" was voiced quickly, along with the immense desire for me to stand by him and help him become the man he was meant to be because of my love. The man who had survived so much tragedy and crazy in his life that only I could fix. No other person on this earth could ever come close to loving me as much as he did. None. And he worked hard to make me believe it while crafting this perfect facade to me and the outside world around him.

My fellow dragon slayers, this is how abuse within relationships begins.

The relationship grows and thrives with love.

The abuse starts off small with tiny little comments here and there. I remember the first time he told me I looked like a slut. We were in Vegas, only a couple of months into our relationship, and I was dressed up for a concert. I came down to meet him in the bar, and he said, "Jesus, Caroline. You look like a whore."

Check out this next part, folks, because I'm about to lay out a pattern of abuse, which only gets worse and repeats over and over and over and over again for the entirety of the relationship.

So when I told him he hurt my feelings, he blamed me. My man told me I was too sensitive, couldn't take a joke, and blew his comment way out of proportion. He was sorry, but if I learned to take a joke better, then this wouldn't be all my fault because right now, we are fighting because I'm too sensitive.

What did I do? I thought, well, maybe I can't take a joke. Maybe I should just go with the flow and not get my feelings hurt. After all, he tells me he loves me all the time, so it must just be me being super sensitive. I decided to just move forward on the date and keep the peace.

What did he do? Offered to buy me a pair of boots because he loved me so much, and we'd be walking a ton in Vegas.

Maybe it seems small to anyone reading this to define abuse as being told I looked like a whore. But it's the start of what was to come and indicative of what survivors face.

Abuse never starts out as abuse. Abuse always begins with love.

The perpetrator has a plan. The plan is evil and calculated with the specific choices to purposefully inflict pain and trauma- and most often blame the survivor for every act of evil in a twisted mind warp of insanity.

As the years unfolded and the abuse grew worse, the dragon was quietly growing new heads and tentacles all without my knowledge or consent.

Telling me I looked like a whore grew to millions of instances of devaluing me and dismantling my entire belief system about myself, happening slowly over the entire relationship. It would include emotional, verbal, financial, and sexual abuse. It would include isolating me from my friends and family. It would include throwing me against walls and spitting in my face in a crowded restaurant.

Ultimately, what made me finally decide to escape him would be the discovery of his efforts to offer me up for sex with strangers, without my knowledge and consent, to people on the internet. Plus, discovering evidence of numerous affairs with men and women in online forums across the United States whenever he traveled for work and in our own home when I traveled.

These acts of evil are where the dragon began for me, and the first dragon head grew from my lack of understanding the level of abuse I was living. It's true- so crazy and true. Most people living in abuse will say the same thing, "I didn't know I was being abused," and that crazy and crazy-making fueled the dragon. Each type of abuse issued created another dragon head.

These dragon heads need a lot of cultivation. The pattern of blaming me for trying to survive the fire-breathing head, telling me the relationship is all bad because of me, apology with no change and then throwing in a love bomb or boots (Ha!) roses, cards, professions of love, begging me to stay, promises of change and cultivating the firm mantra of only my love could make it stop. It took extensive planning and execution for him to be deceitful, and the ugly dragon heads thrive in the deceit patterns.

I traveled for work quite extensively during the relationship. Every day I was gone, he would text and communicate with pictures from him in our home. He would send me texts about how much he missed me. He would make me homemade signs and take selfies holding the signs. "Sweetpea, come back home soon, I love you so much," would be drawn and held in front of him for each picture sent. I would get new ones every day.

What I didn't know and what I didn't find out until after I escaped was that he would actually plan outfits to wear, go around the house, take pictures, save them and change clothes for a new picture. He would gather enough clothing changes, enough different signs, and he created enough different spots in our house to show how much he loved me. Meanwhile, the minute I left, he'd hop on a plane and fly to another city to have one of his random affairs. And in that city, he would send me the saved pictures from our home, as if he was there.

My abuser worked really hard to craft a perfect facade to the outside world. Really hard! I'm not alone in this story. Not by a long shot. It turns out there are dragons all over the damn world. Let's take a world view now of this domestic violence dragon because my story is reflective of the millions of stories worldwide.

Domestic violence is considered an epidemic by the World Health Organization. There are dragon stories of 33% of the female heterosexual population, 10% of the heterosexual male population. Furthermore, in the LGBTQ+ community, 44% of lesbian women and 61% of bisexual women, while 26% of gay men and 37% of bisexual men all have their own dragon to slay. If you lay in the shame of not reporting, these statistics would be even higher! Chances are you may never know who shows up in the world every day, either personally or professionally, hiding mental and physical bruises from their dragon at home.

A slow dismantling of confidence from the inside out, completed by the person who claims love, but then blames you for every problem in the relationship, tendering in an apology with no real change and offers of a love bomb of attention trying to make the entire relationship look like the early days. The person claims to love, looks you in the eye and says, "This is all your fault," and because the dragon heads grow over time, a person trying to survive believes it and stays. Repeat. Repeat. Repeat.

Sounds crazy, right? Right. It is crazy and crazy-making, and it can last in relationships for decades.

The person surviving abuse just keeps trying to get back to those beginning moments- the moments with zero tears and full of hope. The moments of planning and "Sweetpea, let's dream together. What kind of life can we create?" Holding hands, dancing naked in the bedroom, and falling asleep intertwined like pretzels are the foundation where no dragon ever lives; except that it is always present and hiding under the surface.

The dragon heads of domestic violence make it hard to leave. Financial abuse means people often don't have the money to leave. Isolation means by the time a survivor wants to leave, she (or he or they) doesn't have friends or family to confide in the need for help. When kids are involved, it is easier to stay and be psychologically or physically beaten than the fear of sharing custody.

Let's not forget the startling statistic that when people choose to leave, they have a 75% increased chance of being killed in the first three months after escape.

How did I decide to slay this dragon head of "why didn't they just leave?" (Cue the crowd cheering, "Swing away, Caroline. Swing away!")

I created an entire organization called Safe In Harm's Way, which is dedicated to educating everyone about the feelings tied to relationships so that they can recognize abuse earlier and find the community and resources needed to heal as they decide what to do next.

Here is where the magic happens. At Safe In Harm's Way, we receive emails where people suspect someone they know, maybe a family member, co-worker, neighbor, or friend, is being abused. Instead of judging and asking, "Why don't they just leave?" they ask, "How can I help?"

Why, because they've read our website, Facebook, Instagram, Twitter, Spotify, and YouTube (or like you, reading this chapter!), and they get it. They now understand all the dragon heads a person could be fighting, and it is never a simple choice to just leave. In fact, it could be deadly without the right resources in place.

How can you get or give help? There are contacts and resources at the back of this chapter. We need you.

I slay dragons, and my usual lipstick is either peach or red. My favorite heels are about four inches high. But here's the deal- I can't keep raising my sword by myself. I need an army of fellow dragon slayers, and I'd love for you to join me in the revolution. As I tuck my fire-forged sword back in its sling, with the dragon head of "why didn't they just leave" dead at my feet, I need another person to take my place. Ready to swing away at the next layer of abuse so that one day no one will be hiding their wounds from home, but rather stepping forward into the world with zero fear of dragons.

Join us! Pick up your own sword, and let's go change the world!

Caroline Hammond

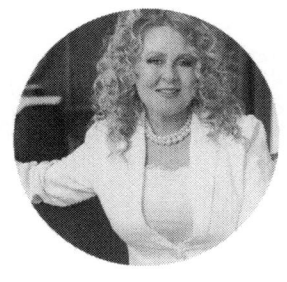

Founder and CEO Safe in Harm's Way

What is Safe In Harm's Way? Let's start with our Founder and CEO, Caroline Markel-Hammond.. The 2020 Boston Scientific Global Volunteer award winner and the Vera Bradley Inspiring Women 2020 award winner has a history of sales, training and presentation success.

As a survivor of domestic violence, plus revival from a death-experience, Caroline uses storytelling to evoke change and has been featured in Forbes, PBS, NPR, partnerships with OAAA, national and regional television, and podcasts as a thought leader in the domestic violence and overcoming adversity arenas, plus international training implementation and curriculum.

https://carolinemarkelhammond.net

https://safeinharmsway.org/

https://ncadv.org/get-help

https://www.thehotline.org/

National Domestic Violence Hotline 1-800-799-7233 (SAFE) or 1-800-787-3224 (TTY)

National Domestic Violence Text Text START to 88788

Reinvention Of a Fat Girl

When I started wanting to have relationships, I had a bit of a confusing start. From my parents I saw a loving one, but the balance of power was off as my Dad got sick and my Mum cared for him - even after she got sick too.

I found it hard to express my needs when I was young because everything was pretty shitty when I went from child to adolescent, money was very tight, and I was continuously bullied at school (and by my sister...) I wanted to be accepted by my Dad's children from his first marriage, but they were mostly adults by the time I came along and already set in their (quite frankly ignorant) ways. The people-pleaser was born from a mixture of this.

I lost my virginity very young, with a guy who said, "if you loved me you would do it," and obviously, I fell for that. My naivety didn't get any better, and that computed in my brain that I should give my body in order to get affection. Already a chubby kid, I began to repeat this pattern that I wasn't good enough because I was fat, so letting a boy feel me up meant I wasn't that gross. Even if it was in secret.

As a teenager, I had two long-term boyfriends. One of which turned out to be gay! I was told later on that if a gay man slept with me, then I must be one heck of a woman. This was told by another gay man who'd struggled to come out when he was young too. Small solace, but it did make me feel a little less rejected (though I didn't find this out until about 5 years later!)

The other boyfriend when I was 17 was just a wet lettuce. He was stuck in permanent "moany git mode," and I didn't want a guy who was more dramatic than me! He had rubbed off on me more than I'd realised. I was on a school trip abroad, a fellow student told me that it was like hanging around a black cloud with me. I'd unintentionally moulded myself into this little goth/emo kid whose natural state was really not to be all doom and gloom. It's safe to say, shortly after this trip, I split up with my boyfriend.

When I went to college to study Performing Arts, I found I could reinvent myself. I could walk away from this perpetually bullied, gloomy goth kid and start to embrace who I wanted to be.

I walked away from being this naive, slightly shy introvert, and I exploded as an extrovert. I did not bloom. This was not a gradual, calm transformation. This was an in-your-face, I'm LOUD AND PROUD HEAR ME ROAR kind of reinvention. I went from 0 - 1000 in a blink.

And with that came the facade. It looked like I was having the time of my life, confident AF and loving everyone, but in reality, I was dying on the inside. I was being the funny fat girl as much as possible during the day, and during the nights, I didn't get almost black-out drunk; I was crying about feeling so shit about myself.

So naturally, I spent a long time being a total slut. I'm ok with that now because I can now look back and realise it was all about my self-worth and not about how I equated physical affection to actual affection.

During my college years, I spent a lot of time bed-hopping, convincing myself I didn't want a relationship, and I was just out to have fun. When in reality, all I wanted was love because I didn't love myself. Any attention was good in my books. So I would sleep around as much as I could, drink a LOT and I convinced myself I was having the BEST time.

Straight after college, I jumped at the chance to go to Greece to work as an entertainer. I reinvented myself once again here. I was this suave performer, who loved life, spoke a bit of Greek, and was ready to constantly party the night away. My love life didn't get much better, but I was starting to get fed up with only having a physical connection rather than an emotional one.

I lasted 1 season in Greece as it was exhausting!

When I came back from my second season as an entertainer in Devon, I was just so done with it all. I was done with the one-night stands, expecting more, done with the heartache and awkward embarrassment of shoving the guy out of the door before work before anyone could see him.

I told my friends I'd had enough, and I actively looked to date rather than go out, get drunk and bring them home.

I met this guy online (this was before the days of dating apps in 2006 - hellooo MySpace), and we hit it off. He was funny, outgoing, had a great group of friends, and he liked me.

I didn't really have many non-negotiables at this point. I was definitely still in the low self-worth stage, and the fact that he liked me put him in a high position.

I stayed with him for a really long time.

I moulded myself to how I thought he wanted me to be. I know you lose yourself sometimes in relationships, and that's exactly what I did.

He knew about my body count, and while he was shocked, he said that didn't matter to him.

The first year or so was fine. But then the cracks started to show.

It started off small. He was a wrestler, so he would wrestle me playfully, but I'd always get hurt in some capacity, then he'd tell me not to be such a baby. There would always be some form of backhanded compliment, and he would constantly say I was not as crazy as his psycho ex. He would bring her up a lot, always derogatory, but then was still friends with her online.

Because I was a performer, I was used to being in the limelight. He was a part-time performer too, and so began the battle for centre stage.

He won. I stepped back. I didn't want him to feel threatened; out came the people pleaser.

Unfortunately, that still wasn't enough.

When we were out with friends, he would constantly comment on my drinking.

I was drinking too much, I was being too loud, too much. I was making a spectacle of myself.

You're not funny, you know.

I found myself at a point in 2008 where I had gone back to University to finish off my degree, then suddenly I lost a family friend, and I just wasn't coping emotionally. I needed him to support me emotionally, but I didn't get it from him. All I got was indifference at best, and there was a constant commentary on my life and how I conducted myself and how much of an embarrassment I was.

It came to a head a couple of months later, we were out in Nottingham for someone's birthday (one of his friends), and I had my elbow grabbed when no one could see, and a vicious whisper in my ear... "Stop fucking drinking. Stop buying shots. Just stop it; you're an embarrassment."

I ignored it and carried on drinking.

He kept on being in my ear, buzzing like a wasp. "Everyone thinks you're a fucking idiot, and you're just being cringe-worthy; stop drinking so much and being so fucking loud, it's so annoying."

That was rich, coming from Mr. LoudMouth himself.

At this point, I'd had enough. My inner rebel was louder than my inner people pleaser. While I didn't say it out loud, I knew my heart was saying, "fuck you, I do what I want." So I did and got blind drunk. We had a huge argument in front of everyone, where he said I'd ruined his friend's birthday and that I was pathetic, and made me apologise to all of his friends - who all looked as awkward AF surrounding me and continued to argue all the way back to the hotel.

I did manage to let him know I was struggling with the fact that my friend had died, but according to him, that made me an attention-seeking victim.

Surprisingly I didn't finish with him that night, but we did take a break about a month later while I was deep in my studies at University, and I went to therapy having cognitive behavioural therapy to help me with depression and the feeling of the world on my shoulders.

It took a further year and a half to split up with him.

During that time, the consistent pattern was this: I still had a huge lack of self-worth. I tried to tell him how I felt, and he would continually zone out or not want to talk, saying it made him feel uncomfortable. He would go on lots of "lads" mini-breaks and constantly neg me (negging was very popular around the release of the book The Game) or downright insult me, but never in front of anyone.

I found my turning point after my Dad passed away. I grieved and spent my summer with my head in the fridge. I found solace in food. So I ballooned to a UK size 26, and my self-worth managed to get even lower than I thought possible.

We went on a holiday with 2 of my friends, and it was then he got caught saying the horrible shit to me he'd so carefully managed to do without people hearing. Now my friends didn't let him get away with that, so once home, I'd had a long chat with my friends, and I had come to the point where I needed to do something.

So I invested in a radical diet to lose weight. I ended up losing over 4 stone (60lbs) in 6 months.

The lack of self-esteem was still very evident, but there had been a turning point in those 6 months.

If I could do that without his support, then maybe I didn't need him around.

We kept the facade up for another 6 months, but by early 2011, I knew it was time. The thing is, he was a coward, treated me like shit because he didn't want to be cast as the bad guy. So I ended it.

He did have the audacity to say when he picked up the last of his stuff that he didn't want me to go back to my old ways. I told him that it wasn't really his place to ask that of me. You have no power over me, bitch.

I didn't "go back" anyway, mainly because I wanted to work on myself.

I came away from the last meeting with him bruised but empowered.

I did work on myself.

I went to America for a face and body art event about 3 months later, on my own (I met a friend out there), and felt amazing.

When I was out with friends about a month after America, I found out he was in the same club as me. We decided to make a sharp exit, but not before I saw this girl dressed up in a toga, looking lovely - I complimented her on her outfit and makeup. She blurted out, "You know I'm <his> girlfriend, right?" I was a bit shocked, but was like, ok...good for you! BYE!

I ended up getting a message from her the very next day, saying that they had split up that night because he was dirty texting another girl and that he'd admitted he'd cheated on me many times during our relationship and did I want to meet up?

Well, of course, I said yes.

When I met her, she was the loveliest, sweetest girl who was so angry that he'd duped her like he had me.

We had the best night, took photos of us together, put them as our profile pictures on Facebook to freak him out. It was hilarious. Yeah, it was also petty as fuck. I didn't really care. I wasn't as upset as I thought I might be about him cheating on me. I even rationalised it... Looking back now, that was totally a learned response, but it spurred me to continue working on myself.

I didn't want to let any guy into my life right then. I needed space, but someone came along who I'd messed around with way back when I was an entertainer in Devon. He was safe. I knew the parameters of our friends with benefits situation. He made me feel sexy, made me feel wanted, and would do almost anything just to make me laugh. He just happened to live halfway across the country, so no real shot at a relationship.

He helped me put myself back together again. I didn't mould myself around him; I was just happy being me for once.

I spent the next year figuring out myself and what I liked to do. I learned to empower myself and push through my own bullshit by using the CBT techniques I learned and my own life experiences. Basically, if it didn't feel right, it wasn't for me. I had started to discover my non-negotiables about what I wanted in a relationship.

I spent the entirety of 2012 and early 2013 working my arse off to save to go travelling. I was working full time, and then weekends face painting or kids' entertainment, I had no time nor inclination for a relationship.

When I went to Australia, it was yet another reinvention. But I wasn't the woman I was back when I exploded onto the college scene over 10 years previously.

I was no longer the people pleaser. I felt like I had a purpose by going to Australia.

This was where I had learned from the past.

I had a mentally abusive relationship under my belt, the loss of a parent and close friend, university, and a lot of general life experience.

I still wasn't at optimum Carla, but I felt more like myself than I ever had. I also had quite a bit of self-worth by this time.

I felt finally I was me in this country. I unleashed my soul, and my happiness found me.

I loved bright threads and to be bright, to be as sunny as the country I was in. I felt at home. I found so much happiness in just being around myself. This is why part of my heart will always be in Australia because this was my grown-up reinvention. This was the biggest one so far, where I became who I am today.

When I did finally come back to the UK, I was much surer of myself. I had real non-negotiables that I wasn't willing to amend for another. I also was still ok with not actively looking for a relationship. I was on tinder (as you do), but there was never anyone who continued to keep my focus until this one dorky guy, who was a nerd like me and had killer dimples.

One date and fireworks in my stomach first kiss later... I knew there was big potential.

AND on the second date, we both laid out our non-negotiables. They were in perfect alignment.

And so... I leapt. Head first into this new relationship. Gone was the ugly bitterness surrounding my ex. Gone was the need to mould myself into something I'm not for another.

It just felt right. It continues to feel right, as we're now married. I'm not saying life is all a bed of roses, but we kept to our non-negotiables for romantic partners and for our lives.

And it works.

The main things I have found since starting this mad journey we call life is this:

- You can't control everything, so if you can't change the situation (as you can't change anyone else but yourself), change the way you feel about it.

- Your partner is not a mind reader. Saying what you want is vital to a balanced life. Same goes for them - you are also not a mind reader!

- Are you an Asker or a Guesser? https://ask.metafilter.com/55153/Whatsthe-middle-ground-between-FU-and-

Welcome#830421 Were you brought up

where it was common to ask, or did you

have to consider all angles until you're

sure it's a yes?

- Talking is good when you preface with
  either of these: Do you want someone to
  just listen or a solution?

- Expressing your needs - what is it you
  want out of life from the other people
  surrounding you, and if you want to grow
  as a person!?

Carla-Jayne Hollingworth

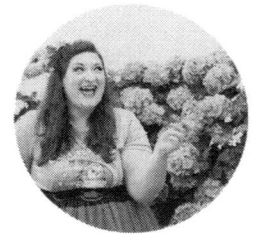 Mindset Mistress, Aggressive Positivity Advocate & Part-Time Mermicorn-Rex

CJ helps frazzled female entrepreneurs overcome hardwired BS beliefs, so that they can be more visible, charge what they're worth and create the ripple effect with their business, without overwhelm or trying to reinvent the wheel.

She stands for being authentic AF and loving what you do with pure passion and is always in your corner to help you get off the self-haterade. www.newleafyourlife.com

https://www.nationaleatingdisorders.org/help-support/contact-helpline

Call 800-931-2237 or Text 800-931-2237

https://www.lifeworkscommunity.com/eating-disorders-treatment/guide-to-uk-free-eating-disorders-helplines

From Surviving to Thriving: The Story of Childhood Sexual Abuse

My story is not a particularly happy story. Nor is it a particularly unique story.

It is a way too fucking common story, which says a lot, for where we are at as a society is on trauma and women and girls and how we treat them. It is also a story that can be fuzzy and jump all over the place - because that is what happens with trauma. Our memories don't form in a nice little linear path, laid out super clearly for us. So when there's jumping around, or when I'm unable to remember specific age-related details, that's just normal for trauma.

What I'm going to talk about does require a trigger warning for sexual abuse. It started when my parents got divorced, which for me came out of the blue. I was around four or five, I think. And suddenly, my dad was just...not there. And that in itself was scary and traumatic.

But that's not the part I want to tell you about.

Imagine for a moment, being 4 or 5, and suddenly, some random man was not only in your house but in your mother's bed. And you discover this by walking into your mom's room first thing in the morning to start your day.

Because that is how I met the man who would become my stepfather and my abuser. In incredibly short order, my mother moved us in with him, and they got married. So he began his free access to me. It started off being very hidden, very secretive.

In my bed when I was sleeping.

In the pool when no one else was around.

In the car when it was just him and I.

I was a child. I was 6. I had no ability to stop him physically or otherwise.

The damage that comes from childhood abuse is not just about the actual abuse. So much of it is about the power differential. The mental and emotional manipulation. The complete loss of control or agency and the game playing that fucks with our developing minds.

Sexual abuse is not just physical; it's mental and emotional abuse at the same time.

I remember trying all kinds of things that my child brain could come up with to try to protect myself—trying not to be alone with him, isolating from family events and spending more time out of the house. But the damn reliance on the adults abusing children allows the abuse to continue.

One of my futile and desperate attempts was to wrap myself up in my blanket and sheet at night before I went to bed, trying to cocoon in as much as I could so that he just wouldn't be able to access me.

His response to that was to take away my fan in the summertime.

We lived in South Africa, and it's fucking hot. And in the summertime, without a fan, it was just unbearable, and I physically could not sleep or tolerate lying wrapped up in so many layers of covering.

And this fucked with me so badly on a mental and emotional level because what my brain understood was that I would be punished for trying to protect myself. Not only that but I would be put in a situation where I had to actively make a choice between being intolerably physically uncomfortable due to the heat or "allow" him access to me.

That manipulation made me a "participant" in my poor, traumatised understanding of events.

Now, as an adult, I can recognise that I held no responsibility whatsoever and that it was all on him. All of it. But it took me a lot of years of healing to be able to recognise that I'd internalised that belief about my participation, stop trying to punish myself for it, and allow the shame to be his.

As is so common with abuse, it escalated from being very hidden to being much more public.

In the pool when my sister, brother, and mother were around. In the hot tub, during family hot tub nights. Right across from my mother. Often while she would be talking to me, looking at me, looking right into my face and eyes. And that fucked with me on so many different levels. What I couldn't understand was how she could NOT see what was happening.

How could I be sitting here and having this vile, terrible thing happen to me by one adult who was supposed to protect and nurture and care for me, while MY MOTHER, the parent who was supposed to be protecting me, keeping me safe and secure was sitting right there, smiling, laughing, chatting away as if for all the world everything was FINE And NORMAL and not doing anything to stop it.

As children, we learn by watching our parents. I learned a couple of really big lessons from this.

1) This was normal.

2) I wasn't worth protecting.

Because, if I was important enough to be protected, then she would have protected me. Right?

If I was better.

If I was worth it.

If I was WHATEVER that was different from who I actually was, then she would protect me, right?

Now both of those were complete bullshit. But that's the thing about warped messages and lessons we learn as kids. Most of them are bullshit, but it doesn't make it any less true in our head, our heart, or our behaviour - until we've unlearned them and replaced them with the truth.

Did you know that it's psychological suicide for us, as children, to acknowledge and admit and understand that the people who are supposed to be caring for us are not capable of it and are instead doing the exact opposite.

Because wrapping our heads around that, as children, means confronting the reality that we are now completely responsible for all of our own needs at an age that we cannot be, at an age that we are biologically programmed to need these adults. And our brains (always trying to protect us, often in very misguided ways) do find a way to keep us psychologically safe by making the only other "logical" assumption.

If they are not the problem. Then we are.

So we internalize the message that it's our fault. Because to do otherwise would break us psychologically. Internalizing the message that it was my fault that it happened in the first place, and then also the message that if I was "worth it" as a child, then my parents would actually do what my parents are supposed to do and take care of me.

When abuse happens at a developmental stage, we internalize so many different messages. Childhood abuse happens at a stage where we're learning about who we are, as individuals, as family members, our place in the world.

And when we learn from trauma, what we learn is low self-esteem, low self-worth, we learn that we are not worth protecting, we learn that we are not worth taking care of, we learn that we do not get to have boundaries, that bad shit happens TO US, that bad shit will always happen TO US.

With sexual abuse, the learning can be very often and was for me, being that our entire purpose as human beings is to meet the sexual needs of the adult.

For so many years as a child, a teen, and as an adult, I wholeheartedly believed that my entire purpose as a human being was dependent on what I could provide sexually for adult men.

And that was my responsibility; that was all that mattered.

We already have such shitty messaging around women and our sexuality in our patriarchal society that our worth comes from what we look like. Our worth comes from what we can provide sexually; our entire existence is contingent upon pleasing men.

My experience compounded that belief, and my behaviour matched. I had no boundaries. I couldn't (physically couldn't due to PTSD responses) say no to men. I equated sex and love and was so desperately looking to be loved, which led to promiscuous behaviour as a teen and adult, which did a fantastic job of reaffirming all of my lower than low self-worth and esteem beliefs I carried about myself.

His abuse had repercussions like ripples in a pond throughout every single area of my life, every single relationship I've ever had and still have, on how I show up in the world, on my mental health and on my physical health. No part of my life or being was left untouched.

It is fucking exhausting at any age. But as a child, to be walking around keeping this giant secret, constantly wondering how no one notices.

Abuse often doesn't get talked about when it happens because there's an overt threat by the abuser. "If you tell, I will do this damage to you, or I will do this terrible, awful thing."

"If you tell, no one will believe you."

In a lot of cases, it's a more covert threat.

The feeling of shame permeates everything because somewhere deep down, you recognise that this isn't okay and that you can't stop it. But everybody's acting like it's okay. So you suck it up, and you shut up about it.

We don't say anything because of that shame. We don't say anything because if we were better, it wouldn't be happening. We don't say anything because if we were worth more, it wouldn't be happening.

And we survive, we exist with the burden of that shame and the burden of the secret and the burden of the responsibility that isn't ours that belongs with the adult, and yet they refuse to take it. And we don't know what else to do. Someone has to carry that, right? And so we do.

Carrying all of that took all of my energy, all of my resources.

This meant, normal, everyday childhood skills and experiences that we have were being missed.

I wasn't learning social skills, I wasn't learning how to interact with other kids, I wasn't learning how to make friends, and I wasn't learning how to be a child.

I wasn't able to be a child because I needed to be a survivor all the time.

And I needed the mental and emotional energy that went into processing it, keeping it secret, managing my feelings around. I didn't have anything left for living.

I got bullied a lot in school. I was already the red-headed kid with the accent. Now I was the awkward, angry, withdrawn, weird red-headed kid with the accent.

I couldn't understand how people couldn't see that there was something terribly, terribly wrong.

All of the very powerful feelings that I had on the inside were so big. It was inconceivable to me that my parents, family friends, teachers, kids at school, even complete strangers simply looking at me couldn't see that SOMETHING was happening.

Surely people had to see the pain.

Surely people had to see the fear.

Surely people had to see just how wrong everything was.

But they didn't. They saw a child "misbehaving." They saw a child who was "acting out," they saw a child who needed punishment, rather than a child who desperately needed adults to be adults and to help.

To this day, I still have remnants of this memory show up in my relationship. I remember stopping what I was doing one day, just standing there, watching my entire family acting as if everything was normal, and everything was fine.

And having this voice screaming in my head, "Why is nobody asking me if I am okay? Why is nobody asking what's wrong? Why won't anybody just ask?"

Nobody ever asked.

It finally became too big a secret to carry for too long a time, and my exhausted, damaged self finally told on him.

It happened because my mother had been diagnosed with cancer, and she was in the hospital.

And I was staying with my dad and my stepmother.

The routine had become for my abuser to pick me up, to take me to the hospital to visit my mom. Creating a situation that worked really well for him because he then had unfettered access to me in the car to and from the hospital.

One morning, my stepmother woke me up and told me to get dressed as he was on his way to pick me up. I don't remember what it was about that morning that was different. Maybe there was nothing different, maybe I'd just reached my threshold. Carrying a secret like this for 5-6 years had taken all I had, and I was done.

Whatever the reason was, I just couldn't do it anymore; I'd hit my breaking point. And I completely lost my shit, I burst into tears, I couldn't speak, I was hysterical. I couldn't say or do anything other than sobbing uncontrollably.

Thankfully someone finally recognised that this wasn't a normal response. And that there was more going on. She closed my bedroom door, leaving me alone, and she called him back and told him he wasn't going to come and get me.

I sobbed for hours, alone in my room. I don't remember writing the note or what I said, but I do remember slipping a note under my stepsister's bedroom door because she was the person I felt most comfortable with voicing anything about it. I couldn't speak about it; the words got stuck in my throat and choked me.

But I could write it down.

My entire life exploded, and every adult in my life handled it in pretty much the worst possible way that they could.

As an adult, I recognise some of them were doing what they thought was right at the moment, but none of it was very trauma-informed or very helpful for an 11 year-old who had just broken the silence about such a huge trauma happening.

It was decided that I needed to confront my abuser in person while at the same time telling my mother what had been happening.

I don't remember having a choice, I don't remember being given the option to say no. I didn't even realise saying no was something I was ever allowed to do with adults.

After my mother came home from the hospital, I found myself sitting in her living room facing her, her husband (my abuser), and her parents.

And trying, amidst hysterical sobbing, overwhelming fear, crushing shame, and debilitating pain, to force the words out, to make them understand.

I don't remember what I said. I don't remember the words that I used or how I phrased them. But I do remember that they didn't believe me.

Predators groom not just their victims but their communities too. They are so good at crafting a persona that radiates false safety and security. They are expert manipulators. It's how they get away with it.

And he was no different. He is, after all, a predator.

My mother looked at me, blinked, stood up, and left the room without a word. I've tried over the years to imagine what was going on in her head. This man that she had brought into our lives, that she was completely dependent on as her cancer progressed, being opted as the worst kind of person you could possibly want around your children.

I learned, years later, that my mother had been a survivor of childhood sexual abuse, but her parents had managed to convince her that she had imagined the whole thing. I'm pretty sure that impacted her response too. It doesn't really matter; the end result was that I didn't have a mother who protected or believed me.

I don't remember ever talking to my mother about it again. Shortly after this happened, she moved back to Canada because she was sick, and she wanted to be near her parents and her family.

And I ended up staying with my dad and my stepmom. That was yet another layer of trauma and abandonment, fear and pain, and a massive mindfuck for a pre-teen. I didn't want to go with them, I didn't want to be anywhere near my abuser, and I wanted my mother to choose me, but she had chosen him and left.

And that was an event that further stamped those shitty beliefs about myself into my very core as a human being. People in my life who should fight for me, we're not going to. People in my life who should care for me, we're not going to.

We are taught by society and biologically, that our mothers are the ones that we should be able to rely on; they are the ones who will go mama bear and protect their children. And that's not always true.

I am still working through unresolved grief and anger at her.

My mother's mother's response was to try and convince me that I'd misunderstood his intentions and that it hadn't happened. Hey, it worked for her once, so she stuck with it. And my mother's father's response was to attack and shame me, to tell me that it was unacceptable that I was causing this much trouble and that I was breaking up the family.

I've already tried to help you understand how damaging the abuse was to my life. There are times where I still wonder if the lack of support, the lack of understanding and belief, the lack of protection and care, the lack of human decency extended to me by my "family" when I came out with this big secret was more traumatic and more damaging.

Because it, too, taught me a lot of things.

Not to ask for help. Asking for help was dangerous; there was no fucking point to it, and it made things worse. It taught me that I was not believable, which had the very common knock-on effect that when I was raped as a teenager and as an adult, I didn't tell anybody about it for years because of that exact lesson. Just don't tell because there's no point to it. And the pain that you will go through is not worth it.

It taught me that family cannot be trusted.

It taught me that adults cannot be trusted.

It taught me that people cannot be trusted.

And that is something that I still struggle a lot with. It's better; it's infinitely better. Those trust issues no longer rule my life or decision-making or behaviour.

But they still show up. And I still have to remind myself that it's not true of all people. And I still have to use the tools that I have learned in therapy over the years to talk about hard things and to reach out for and to ask for help and connection when I need it.

It took me a lot of years to get here; to get out of the darkness, to heal and move through the anger, to release the shame, and to let it be his to carry. Decades of my adult life were spent just putting one foot in front of the other, trying to survive one more day, one more hour, one more minute some days. It impacted my personal and business relationships.

Lost in a place of low self-worth and not believing that I was allowed to be happy, to find love.

To have a career that I wanted and to make the money that I wanted to. My core beliefs about myself were that I existed as an emotional, mental and physical garbage disposal, and everybody else was going to land on me.

And I accepted that, which came with accepting that kind of behaviour from others and from myself. And I spent decades in a place of anger; anger that it had happened. Constantly trying to figure out why it had happened to ME. Anger that covered up pain and fear. Because it wasn't fair, it wasn't okay that it happened. But I spent so much time stuck in that place of focusing on it being not okay and not fair that I didn't do my healing.

One of the most painful lessons I learned was that while the fact that it happened wasn't my fault, the emotions and the fallout from it became my responsibility because that's just the reality of the world. As unfucking fair as that is, I spent so much time trying to avoid that truth that I hindered my own healing, and I made things a lot worse for myself by resisting the pain and trying to avoid the pain rather than healing from the pain.

When I finally got to a place of not having enough emotional energy to continue resisting and just wanting to move through it and actually doing my trauma healing, everything fucking changed. And here's what I now know to be true about myself; I'm a survivor, I'm a fighter, and I was made for great things; it just took me a little longer to recognise that.

I fought Every Fucking Day. And I kept fighting. I've been in therapy since I was 11 years old. It took decades, it took pain, and It took time. It took fucking it up a lot. But now, I have turned all of the shit that I have been through, that I have survived, into something that is helping hundreds of women.

Now, I work with women who are on their own healing journey.

I get to be, for them, the person that I needed that wasn't available for me, as a child or as an adult. I work with women who need access to information and support because they don't have that in their own life. Women who have done the most incredible things, and who have built the most incredible fucking businesses against the most incredible odds. And they've done it anyway, just like I did, and they now have that safe place to go and unpack the things that they need to really move through and heal.

I took the shit, the pain, the fear, the PTSD responses, the awfulness, and I made meaning out of it and I did that intentionally because I refuse to allow him to have any kind of power or control of my life anymore, I changed my life, and now I help other women change theirs.

The reward of seeing their healing and growth is so powerful, and for me, it has become one of the most healing things. As I work with my clients and I allow them the space to heal, my healing continues.

Because here's the thing that I believe about healing, we're never fully done. We don't reach a point where we have nothing else to work on ever again; it's an ongoing process. As we learn and grow and heal, we uncover other layers, and that's just part of life, and that is what brings peace, joy, contentment, freedom, and power.

Erin Moore

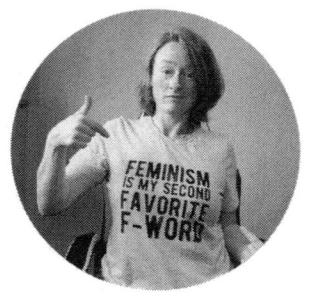

Owner of Authentic AF Coaching

Erin is a trauma informed business, mindset and coach.

She has built 2 x 6 figure businesses while healing from a shit ton of compounded trauma, and has been helping female entrepreneurs do the same for years.

Erin has worked with many female business owners who have gone from struggling with their self worth and shitty internal messaging and conditioning to confidently building business empires in as little as 6 - 12 months.

She started this business because she was sick & tired of women struggling with self worth, fear, boundaries, shitty relationships, impostor syndrome and not being able to find a solution that both supported and uplifted them while kicking their ass into gear, with love. And if you haven't noticed, she swears a lot too.

erin@authenticafcoaching.com

https://www.rainn.org/

National Sexual Assault Hotline. Free.

Confidential 800-656-HOPE

https://www.rcne.com/links/sources-of-help-for-survivors/

The Art of Starting Over

Women from our (South Asian) culture think American women have it all. We think you can do whatever you want to do with your career or life and also that you are not 'answerable' to anyone. Meaning you don't need approval or validation. On the other hand, we (women from 3rd world countries) are expected to be 'submissive.'

Anyway, I was of the opinion that women in first world countries don't need to be submissive. They're not oppressed, and they can do whatever they want to do, they can become whatever they want to become. You can be different, diverse, and celebrated all at the same time.

I moved to the US in 1996, and I started to see that women of the first world countries don't have it all; you have almost the same issues we do (in our part of the world). Maybe not as big, but you have the same issues. The U.S is called the "**Land of Opportunity** where one could achieve anything they put their mind to, no matter who they are." So I was thinking, yes, I'm moving to the US! I have a master's degree, and I wanted to do a Ph.D., make this world a better place by serving its people, and so much more! I thought to myself, I'm going to the land of opportunities, and I'm going to make my dreams come true. Little did I know that life doesn't work like that. It doesn't just grant you your wish, just because you wished for it. There is ALWAYS a price to pay, sacrifices to be made, and not to mention overcoming obstacles, frustrations, and failures without losing focus from your goal. You see, I came from a privileged background to the point that people used to call me spoiled and proud. I had not seen or experienced the 'actual struggle.' So I was totally oblivious to it.

You see, we all have to start somewhere. Some of you, like me, may have had multiple starts. The US is where my multiple starts started. I was thinking that with higher studies, I could pursue my dreams. I didn't think being married would be an obstacle in my way. Because of all the responsibilities I had, it was hard to study further. I knew I could either pursue my dreams or be the submissive wife I was supposed to be. I even tried being submissive because that's what's expected of me. You're supposed to make your home and make sure everyone else is happy. I took the older women of my family's advice and tried to focus on home and family, and sacrificed my dream.

I tried, but I failed. It was not the 'real' me. People didn't understand, and they would ask me, "why are you so rebellious?" They would say, "you're like this black sheep of the family," and they wanted nothing to do with me because of who I was as a woman. As a woman, I am supposed to just take care of everyone around me. But I couldn't do justice to my responsibilities at the cost of my ambitions and dreams.

So here I was with yet another 'start' after I ended my marriage. New country, new people, new language that I could speak, but a whole new culture as well. Neighborhoods, cities, everything was new.

But money buys you choices. I figured if I had money, I would be able to make different choices. So that was the only thing that was on my mind. I was going to make a lot of money. And that's it. I could help others and pursue my dreams later.

I was in survival mode.

So I focused on taking care of my son and making enough money to 'start' yet again. But guess what, I didn't realize I checked all the boxes of being a brown, Muslim, divorced woman. And that meant working as a cashier (remember, this was the 90s)

I had confidence; that was not the problem. The problem was I was emotionally and mentally shattered. Nobody understood me. All they could think of was to marry me off to someone else right away. I felt like I went backwards.

Spending two years in my marriage took me six years back.

However, I didn't give up, and I didn't care what people thought of me. All I wanted was to get a job that would provide me and my son a comfortable lifestyle. Remember I said I had the confidence, I had the degree, but I also checked all the boxes of being a brown, Muslim, divorced woman.

Anyway, to make a long story short, I did get a decent job and for which I worked really hard and made my way up. Yes, there were income gaps at that time, but I didn't care about that.

I didn't want to raise my voice, and I didn't want to do anything that I didn't have time for. I didn't have time to worry about something that was going to slow me down. If I raised my voice then,

I would have been too much of a problem. That was stressful. I was by myself, so I just moved on.

I learned that my assistant was being paid the same as I was, so I just started applying to different jobs. I went in a different direction with another company that was more diverse. So I wasn't fighting for my income or income equality because I'm a woman, a woman of color, plus my religion, and it was post 9/11.

The world after 9/11 was very different from the people from my religion and my culture. And to top it off, my last name is Khan. So you can very well imagine I was into this explanatory mode at all times. I had to explain myself to so many people that I didn't do it (9-11). But then people perceived me poorly anyway because I came from "over there" that I belonged "there," and those are my people.

That hurt really bad at times. Because I consider this my country, and all I wanted to do was to pursue my dreams and provide a comfortable lifestyle for my son. So income gap, racism due to my color, my religion, or my marital status, it all didn't matter to me at that time.

People were wondering how I was climbing the corporate ladder and not flipping burgers. I was very close to making six figures back in 2003. It was the first year I was going to make six figures, and guess what happened, I lost my job.

I lost it all just like that because of some politics in the office. Oh, and did I mention I checked all the boxes of being a woman of color, Muslim and divorced? And you guessed it right, I had to 'start' again.

There I was in New York with my last name as Khan, my skin color as brown, and my religion as Islam. As if that wasn't enough, I developed health issues. I mean, why wouldn't I?

I was forced to choose between taking care of my health(back issue) or work. If I didn't make money because I was sick, then who was going to take care of me and my child? I started looking for anything I could do while staying in bed because my back was so bad. I was bedridden for months. I thought to myself, what could I do to make money while completely being bedridden in 2003?

Nobody was thinking like that. We didn't have remote work then. We didn't have freelancing.

We had nothing that we have today. So I was trying to figure out what I could do to pay my bills when I couldn't even get out of bed. Who was going to hire me?

That's when I realized I could translate because I know three languages. Back in the day, they didn't have these translation apps. I said this is my perfect formula. I'm going to be in my bed providing translation services from my computer, except there was one problem.

Nobody wanted to hire me.

I don't know if it was my color, my last name, or my religion, you will not believe when I was hired at, what were the terms of my pay? I was making about $45 to $48 an hour before I got fired. I was hired by a gentleman (who I still have a lot of gratitude for the opportunity) for .33 cents an hour. That's not even $1 an hour! However, since this was yet another 'start' from scratch. I took it because I got to work from home. That was the whole plan.

I worked all week, 12 hours a day. You know how much one paycheck would be for one week? $7. But I had to make it happen. I could have gotten stuck saying, "why is this happening to me." Is this because of my color, or that I am a woman, my religion? I didn't have time for that.

I had to survive.

So I did that job, and then I hired somebody else to do that job because for them making 33 cents an hour was a big deal. I started sending proposals to other companies for translation services, and I got hired to do translation for two separate companies, each at $1200 a month.

$2400 should be enough, I thought. But my goal was to make six figures. And guess what? In three years, I reached my six figure goal from starting at 33 cents an hour.

So that was my third time 'starting' over, emotionally and financially, starting life again. Until one day, I found out that the interns I was working with were being paid more than I was. I was flabbergasted. Actually, that would be a small word to describe how I felt at that time. I didn't know what to say. So I didn't say anything, and as usual, I removed myself from that team, that company, quietly. I told myself, I have got to go on. I felt alone.

I wasn't going to start a movement there; they would look at me like I was crazy. They would just see me as ungrateful. But I was grateful for what I was doing, but companies can't be so unfair that interns are making more than a supervisor.

I started again, from zero, from scratch, and started my own business. It took me about two years to get the hang of everything and put systems in place, and do the stuff to make automation happen.

Then the pandemic happened. I lost my clients, so I changed the direction of my business and created new offers. You guessed it right; this was yet again, another 'start.'

I tell people I have had multiple starts, and every 'start' required a different version of me.

Every start was harder than the last start, both emotionally and financially. I'm not growing any younger. Now my kids are older, so I don't have to worry as much about them. So when I was forced to start again due to the pandemic, I chose to teach others what I have learned all these years from working from home, totally online.

I am doing very well. Allahumdulilah

I cannot thank the Almighty enough for all the blessings.

So what if I was not the normal submissive person? So what if I was the black sheep of the family? So what if I made mistakes? "It takes strength to fit in, and it takes courage to stand out." And every 'start' just required a stronger Nosheen, reminding myself to take this one last tiny scary step each day.

Like this chapter you are reading, this too is part of yet another 'start,' yet another scary step towards authorship :)

Be the black sheep of your family!

Do the scary thing every day!

It has brought me this far, and it'll take you far as well. Just start!

Nosheen Khan

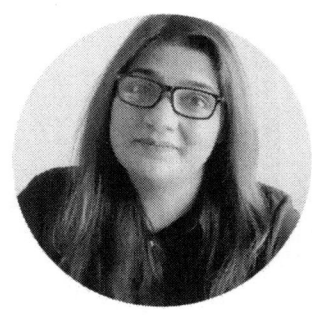

CEO of Automate To Accelerate

Automate tasks so you can make more money while spending less time in your business. Let me help you preserve creative energy, get more done, reach more people, bring in more revenue without the burnout and missed opportunities!

EasySalesAutomation.com

https://nisahelpline.com/

888-315-NISA (6472)

https://therapyformuslims.com/hotlines/

Moms Need Boundaries Too

The whole shitstorm started on December fifth, 2015. My daughter was in an IHSA Horse Show. She was representing her high school. And in IHSA shows, you draw a horse. You don't get to ride your own horse, you ride a random horse. The horse she was on got spooked, she fell off the horse and hit her head. The emergency medical service, EMS at the scene, cleared her to return because they didn't see any problems. She climbed back up into the saddle, finished the horse show, and did well.

Texting me from her boarding school that night, she sent, "Hey, Mom, I fell off the horse today, and I bumped my head. It was no big deal. I'm fine. Everything's okay."

A couple of days later, I got a call from the nurse at the school saying, "Hey, we've got Laura in the infirmary, and she's acting a little drowsy and woozy." I responded, "Okay, that could be typical for a concussion; let her rest." We discussed whether to take her to the emergency room. Chances were that they could only do a CT scan. Unless you think she's got broken bones in her head or another obvious head injury, there's nothing anyone can do- concussions are weird that way. We understood that we'd need her to see a neurologist or a head injury specialist if she was still symptomatic when she came home.

A week went by, and it was time for her to come home for Christmas break. My Au Pair went to pick her up from the airport. Laura is standing there on the curb, waiting. She gets into the car with the Au Pair and the other kids. Laura lost her cell phone. She'd forgotten her credit card. You'd ask her a question, and you would get a confusing, unrelated answer. Her brain wasn't right. It was literally like being in Alice in Wonderland, talking to the Mad Hatter, not Laura. When the Au Pair brought her home, we weren't sure what to do because every time we'd ask her a question, we'd get another nonsensical answer. For a while, she wasn't sleeping. Without warning, she wasn't awake. She certainly was all over the place. After about 24 hours, we took her to the emergency room at the University of North Carolina at Chapel Hill's Medical School- UNC- and asked them what the hell was wrong with our daughter. They were uncertain about the extent of her injury, but she was showing signs of a concussion. So they admitted her to UNC hospital, and they did every test known to man; spinal taps, an MRI. They tested everything, and they couldn't find anything except a traumatic brain injury. The signs of a traumatic brain injury don't show up on an MRI. It was the only answer that they had left to explain any of her symptoms. They could definitely see that when they did the spinal tap, she got better. It was obvious there was an issue, possibly pressure on her brain from the head injury. Since it was three days before Christmas, they sent her home with no follow-ups.

Fast forward a couple of weeks; she seemed to appear to be getting a bit better. We had a neuropsych evaluation, which she completely failed. She couldn't answer any of the questions. Her brain was totally mush. We thought maybe the structure of being back in boarding school would help because she would have to get up and go to bed at certain times. Follow a familiar routine. Students have to do certain things at certain times in certain places. We removed her from most of her classes, so she could just be herself in her favorite environment. After three days, the school called us, "Hey, you need to come and get Laura, she is not acting normal." We now realized there were delusions. For example, Laura thought the inspirational speaker they had at the school for a presentation was talking directly to her. She thought the girls in the hall were talking about her, and she was hearing voices. So I drove back up to Pennsylvania from North Carolina, and we packed everything out of her dorm room and then shipped everything else home. And thus began our new life. It was the middle of Girl Scout cookie season; I had 10,000 boxes of Girl

Scout cookies in the garage. I was leading four troops. One mother decided on the same day that I was retrieving Laura from Pennsylvania that she had to come and bang on the front door and demand that my husband takes her cookie money. She got really upset when he was short with her. Two weeks later, I got a lecture from the council to be nicer to people. That also coincided with Laura's next hospitalization. She came to us on Valentine's night and shared her thoughts, "Dad, Mom, I'm thinking about setting myself on fire."

We immediately took her back to the hospital. She was in the emergency room for 24 hours, similar to many people who have suicidal ideations. There just are not enough beds to go around for the number of patients in crisis. They eventually moved her into a pediatric unit because she was 17. One doctor said they weren't sure; maybe it was schizophrenia. They couldn't get her stable. Her medical team couldn't figure out the right mix of medications to work or how it was going to work or any of it. They eventually found a combination of medications that seemed to work okay enough for her. However, the risk was that she could seem to be perfectly stable and then flip at the drop of a hat to become suicidal. They released her to come home with little follow-up again, as is typical in our mental health system, so she needed 24/7 supervision, which meant that we couldn't even leave her at home alone. She couldn't be anywhere by herself at all. We had to supervise everything she did. This situation dragged on for the next two years.

My life as I knew it was unraveling by this point. I had my home care agency; the Women's

Entrepreneur Network- My Facebook group- was growing into something big; I was doing some business coaching and consulting. I was taking her to every single meeting with me, taking her to work with me every day. She became my shadow, a constant by my side. The next year I started having what seemed to be heart attack symptoms. This landed me in the emergency room, which I took as a warning. I couldn't let things keep going on as they were. I had to make some tough decisions. So, I let my home care agency go; I sold it for what I could get for it. I pulled everything in and decided that I would just do business consulting and work on social media. No building websites, not yet, because it would be too much for me to handle. My whole life imploded because of the escalating situation, because of everything that happened.

It shot our finances to hell. My home care agency was no longer a source of income. Laura's multiple trips to the hospital and subsequent ongoing medical bills were adding to the financial strain on our family. I had debts left from the business, and the medical bills needed to be settled, so I started the procedure of filing for bankruptcy.

My husband hit the roof. "She's faking it. She's playing you." Over the next few months, I started driving for Uber when I didn't have my shadow with me. At night, I would go driving, and during the day, I had her. There was a gradual improvement from her medication. My business grew at a painful and lethargic pace. Things seemed to be okay. She even got a part-time job in senior care, which was a step towards her former career path. She always dreamed of becoming a nurse. In December of that year, we were taking her back and forth to her job because she couldn't drive just yet. Things seemed to improve. Then, in September 2017, she went off of all of her medications, cold turkey. We didn't realize what she did at first.

For a while, things seemed to be just fine. In retrospect, it looked like she was having a manic episode. But she was working. She was okay. She was cooking. Laura was doing most of the things that you would expect a young adult to be doing at 19. We got her back into school. Everything looked great on the surface.

In March 2018, I was running a virtual summit. On the day the summit started, she wasn't feeling well. We realized she was in the middle of having another psychotic break and another psychotic episode. She had an additional occurrence of catatonia, which is highly correlated with schizophrenia. Basically, the patient loses the ability to control their speech, their body, their reactions, and they go into this very delayed reaction mode. If you asked her a question, it could take her minutes to respond.

Once we saw that happening, we got her back into the hospital. They kept her at Duke for about a week, and then they discharged her in the middle of the summit. To say that it impacted my business would be a colossal understatement. Trying to promote a summit with a kid going in and out of the hospital was not really conducive to running a successful event. A few thousand people signed up, which was short of our goals based on the reach that we had. She was discharged, admitted, and discharged. They admitted her with many suicidal ideations. What's clear now is that she was suffering from psychosis. I was trying to balance kids and work and driving for Uber and growing a business and serving clients. It was a three-ring circus. She, at that point, just became incredibly unstable. Laura had flunked out of school. They had removed her from the adult High School Program at Wake Tech for non-completion of her course. She didn't have any clean underwear at the hospital; the doctors wanted us to go out and buy her new clothing. We refused, saying, "No, she's got at least 96 pairs of underwear at home." She had been spending all of her paychecks on more and more and more stuff and things and clothing. She completely overfilled her room. After multiple hospitalizations and one extended hospitalization, it was time to send her to the state psychiatric hospital.

The state psychiatric hospital is really hard to get into. But it's generally designed for long-term stays and for patients that are incredibly difficult to stabilize or not able to stabilize at all. We told them she couldn't come home because she was so unstable. The thing you have to realize is people don't just get hospitalized; they have to be actively a threat to themselves or others in order to be hospitalized at a state psychiatric hospital. The inpatients have to be a suicide risk or a homicide risk. They kept her in the state hospital for a few more months. After they discharged her, only six weeks later, she attempted suicide by overdose. I called 911. An ambulance was in the driveway. The police showed up. My younger daughter drove home from school because she needed to change her clothes. She walked in on her sister being carted out. It was divine timing. I don't know how she figured out which of the medications my daughter had overdosed on, but she did. She also retrieved all of her older sister's browser history and social media history, showing us what she had been researching prior to her suicide attempt. They kept her in the hospital for another seven weeks and discharged her a couple of days before Thanksgiving. Meanwhile, we were trying to keep the other kids' lives as normal as we could. Normal being a relative term. Just keep everybody going. Keep swimming.

They released her from the hospital, this time on a new medication for about three months. What we didn't realize was that the new medication would introduce a whole new level of delusions, homicidal ideations, and plans—resulting in multiple hospitalizations. Laura told the staff that she was homicidal, but she never told us she was homicidal. In July of the following year, I made my health a priority. I scheduled my bariatric surgery, and she decided she was suicidal the day before my procedure. So I dropped her off at the emergency department again the day before my surgery.

What do my children do when the next thing happens with Laura? They call me when I am in recovery. In a way, it was a relief to instruct my other children, "Hey, y'all need to call Dad. I'm going to be out of commission while I am recovering here for three weeks." So my husband got to deal with Laura for a brief period, and it was eye-opening for him. But later in July, her longtime childhood friend messaged me, "I think you need to get Laura to the hospital." I typed, "What's up?" Victoria texted, "Laura is really not right. And she's thinking about killing you guys." I asked if she could give me the screenshots of her messages, and she sent me all of them. Then we called 911 for EMS. She confirmed to them she was homicidal. We tracked and figured out which of the delusions corresponded to which particular thought pattern because she cooperated.

She's incredibly brilliant. She presents different personas to different people, different delusions, at different times. They eventually admitted her to the University of North Carolina- Chapel Hill hospital, where she spent another two weeks in the ER waiting for a bed and in a hospital out on the coast. We put her on the waitlist for our state psychiatric hospital, but the insurance company insisted on having her discharged. The insurance company agreed to have her put into a program. Three days into the day program, they discharged her for basically being too psychotic and upsetting the other patients in the partial hospitalization program. While all of this was happening, I started building websites; I was seeing clients and making progress. I had given up Uber by that point, about a year before. I'm building my business ever so slowly, ever so carefully, bit by bit.

People were asking me why my business wasn't growing faster. Why I wasn't making money hand over fist. I spent half my time dealing with doctors and hospitals and social workers managing all the medical side of things while building websites and doing social media management, and trying to grow a team. It's been a kind of long, slow slog that way. There were more hospitalizations between the hospital and the emergency room. Two weeks in the emergency room here, a week in the emergency room there, waiting for a bed. We were on a first-name basis with most of the police officers in our town. We were lucky. I attribute some of our treatment to the fact that we are white and we live in a very affluent neighborhood. Had the situation been any different, making those kinds of calls about having a child with homicidal ideations, I'm pretty sure things would have ended up quite differently. Ultimately, she ended up in another hospital here locally whose social worker basically said, look, we're trying to get her to the state psychiatric hospital for a long-term hospitalization, but she keeps not getting all the way up the waitlist. Your best option is to just drive her there yourself. We're going to discharge her because insurance is going to make us discharge her before she's really ready. You need to take her to Central Regional Hospital, CRH. Preferably after giving her a few hours at home to have cause to have her hospitalized again, and then take her to CRH. So we did; we brought her home for 16 hours, the shortest time at home with her between hospital stays... We took her back to CRH, and the doctors there were aghast. It was almost like they were expecting us. "Well, Laura, we've seen your name on the waitlist." The admitting doctors told us they didn't expect her to get completely stable at this point. I didn't either, because that's how psychosis is. Once you've been in psychosis for over six months, you never come back out. It's not reversible. At that point, and with our level of medical knowledge, we needed a group home. She couldn't come home because she had active homicidal ideations- and a plan to kill us. Those won't go away.

Some days can be better than others. On the better days, her impulse control is okay. After finding the hidden stash of knives, blades, scissors, and sharps in her room, from when she had an active plan to kill us, I don't think that it's the best choice for us or for any of her siblings for her to come home. So they admitted her in November 2019, just before COVID hit. I found some amazing social workers. They came out of nowhere, we were not in the hospital system; we were out of our element. It forced us into becoming experts on finding people who were familiar with how the mental health system works. Those who shared tips and tricks were an immense resource to get her funding set up for a group home. They walked me through the process. Since we were in the middle of COVID, we had plenty of time in the hospital because they couldn't discharge her without a safe discharge plan. We would not accept the option of bringing her home for obvious reasons. The situation gave us plenty of time to locate the proper placement and funding, which thankfully has come through. It's been amazing. My other kids got to spend time together. During COVID, I found out that my older son is quite a baker; he really enjoys baking. And we made thousands of cinnamon rolls together. It was a perfect time to work on growing an online business. It's been an excruciating struggle, but we might be on the other side of it now. Things are looking up. She's in a group home, and it's a team effort to keep things under control. But we're managing, and I'm excited to be on the other side of the shitstorm.

Haley Gray

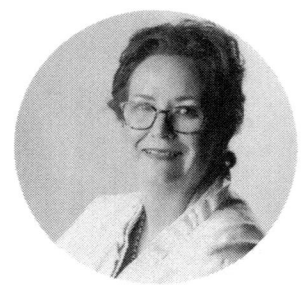

Founder Women's Entreprenuers Network

Haley Lynn Gray is a #1 international best selling author, keynote speaker, and marketing strategist. She is the founder of Women's Entrepreneur Network and Fiercely Marketing. She is passionate about helping small business owners grow their businesses creatively and on a budget.

There is no one size fits all for leadership or business modeling. We are all unique, so playing to our strengths yields the best outcomes.

She is the mother of four active kids, and has a mini zoo in her home, with a variety of pets including cats, a dog, a horse, rabbit, fish, and turtles! She understands that sometimes life gets in the way and is messy, but that it is beautiful anyway.

http://fiercelymarketing.com

https://www.nami.org/home

https://www.adolescenthealth.org/Resources/Cl

inical-Care-Resources/Mental-Health/Mental-

Health-Resources-For-Parents-of-

Adolescents.aspx

Oh God, I'm Gay

I remember when I realized I was a lesbian. I asked God for this not to be the case, much like the stories in the Bible of Jesus asking for the cup to pass from Him, but knew I too couldn't escape my fate. The thought I had was, *Oh, God, I'm gay.* I was 14-years-old and had developed a crush on a teacher, a female teacher. I had reflected on the fact that my friends were all talking about boys in school. I didn't really care because we had grown up with them all. I came from a small town and didn't see them any differently than in the 8th grade as I had in the 1st or 2nd. But I saw girls differently. I was also jealous of the fact that they wanted to go out with these guys and not bring friends like me along.

In that reflection, *Oh, God, I'm gay*, I realized I didn't know what to do with that.

This was a time before anything gay was on television. There were no sitcoms or dramas about gay people. The only movie I found with lesbians in it back then was *The Hunger* with Susan Sarandon, Catherine Deneuve, and David Bowie. It was a vampire horror movie in which Deneuve played a head vampire that was bisexual. She was with David Bowie at the beginning of the movie, and she ended up with Susan Sarandon by the end. I don't remember how in the world I got a copy of that movie, but I did and hid it under my bed. As I grew older, I tested my bravery by ordering a few books by lesbians that I didn't think my parents would recognize the titles of and would also hide those books under my bed. I tried underground efforts like a spy to figure out who I was.

At the same time, I was trying to be successful in school, becoming Sophomore Class President, Junior Class Vice President, and Senior Class President. I found being in front of my classmates and showing out was something that I enjoyed. It led to my eventual profession. At the time, I used it as a cover up as well. The beauty of being in a small town that was very Protestant-based was I could feign virginity and say I didn't want to lose that before I got married. The guys really didn't give me a hard time about having sex. So I was able, as a woman, to get away with it. I can't imagine what it's like for my male counterparts in that arena. But at least for women, they weren't expected to have sex that young in my hometown. So I did not have sex with a man.

My sophomore year in high school, I got to know a junior who I remember thinking was very pretty in the previous yearbook. I can't remember how we got to know each other, but we became friends. Then we became lovers. She and I were together for about nine months, secretly. And we would coordinate times to get out of class at the same time so we could meet in the bathroom just to have a moment of affection. The good thing about being the same gender is that when you have someone spend the night with you, you're able to be together, have a night together, as long as you're quiet and don't let your parents hear. We were in love. She would write me love letters, and I would do the same.

There was a prom in which she invited a guy to prom, and I invited a guy to prom, and we went on a double date. That was the way we got to go to prom together. It was hard but at the same time exhilarating to be able to do it.

Then things changed. She fell out of love with me and fell in love with a guy. So I had to experience her being able to be in public with a guy and me not being able to share my honest emotion in public about that because she was still supposed to be my best friend. That's what everybody thought. So I had to really hide how I felt to keep up that public persona of supporting her, even though it broke my heart to watch her be able to be out in public with this guy. It's just a lonely experience to be gay and in the closet.

When I was in high school as a lesbian, it was the 80s, and it was the time of AIDS. And aids was a "gay cancer." They had not figured out it was a virus or something that straight people could have as well. There was a blood drive in my high school, and I was one of the class officers. It was my job to coordinate it and to get everything in order. One thing the Red Cross had set up was a room divider where a survey was provided. There was a card that had your name on it and asked a simple question, should we use your blood? Yes or no? The reason was so anyone who was a drug user or gay could let them know not to use their blood. This way, you didn't have to tell anybody you knew or expose yourself. As a lesbian, I wasn't sure what that meant for me because it's "gay cancer." They knew men were getting it for the most part, but there was no information about lesbians.

So I chose to not even give blood. I offered the excuse that as Class President, I was just too busy that I didn't want to get lightheaded. I didn't want to compromise myself in order to do my job. But it really was about me hiding the fact that I was a lesbian and not sure what they should do with my blood. There was a lot of confusion at the time. Again, it's a case where I was raised in a Protestant environment. I was afraid my parents would reject me. I was afraid my siblings would reject me. I was afraid God was punishing me. And there was no information.

I used to love school, elementary, and junior high school. High school was miserable for me because everybody was dating. Couples were revered in this very political environment, and I dated guys as a cover. That was not fair to them, and it was not fair to me. I wish I could have been honest with the guys; I wish I could have found a gay guy that I could have had as a partner in crime. Even though I'd slept with a woman, she was now with a guy, and I felt like I was the only lesbian in the world. When you're lying about something, you feel very isolated. And again, there was no representation on television.

When I went to college, I decided I was not going to deal with it. I attended the University of Tennessee and committed to having fun with friends and forget dating. For most people, college is the time where they have sexual adventures, but for me, sex equated to just being resentful, lonely, confused, and not something that was freeing. It was something that was very isolating. I spent most of my time with friends who were focused more on school stuff and attending ball games.

In hindsight, it is a very sad thing that during my high school and college years, sex was not something that was fun. I graduated from the University of Tennessee, but before I did, I met somebody. The last semester of my senior year, I went to gay clubs in Atlanta, which was about a three-hour drive from Knoxville. It was time for me to get back out in the world and go somewhere away from home that was safe. I finally felt a lot freer sexually and made up for lost time with women in Atlanta, where I moved after school.

I got a job at Turner Broadcasting and was still in the closet. I realized then that people are in the closet because their parents don't know it. Because here I am in Atlanta, far from college, far from high school, far from the people that I was worried about, and yet still felt the need not to be out, and that was because of my family.

I later worked at a local bookstore called Oxford. It was a very progressive environment and one of the first bookstores in the country to have its own coffee shop. It had an African-American section, a Gay & Lesbian section, a Native American section, and many others. This was back in the early 90s before Barnes & Noble ever thought about having those kinds of areas in their bookstore. I met gays and lesbians and straight people and bisexuals who all worked there. I realized then when they didn't react or get surprised when I said I was a lesbian, that I could live a normal life and be out.

I decided to come out to my family. I was tired of lying. I was tired of feeling the way I felt. I was afraid that my family would reject me but thought if they do, they do. At least I would be out and could be who I am. I could be with somebody in public and be proud of the relationship I was a part of. I thought I'd try a sibling first. My brother came to Atlanta to see me. We were sitting on the couch, and I was nervous. I finally said,

"Well, I've got something to tell you."

"What is it?"

"I'm gay."

"Well, tell me something I don't already know."

I laughed out loud. All the tension just melted into the floor. He didn't care. I didn't have to go to my sister because he got to her first. She sent me this heartfelt letter to express how she accepted me for who I was. It still brings tears even after 30 years.

The one I talked to was my mother, and she just wanted me to be happy. It was my father that I was really intimidated by. He was a six foot two, an ex-military officer who was a star basketball player, total alpha male who was a devout Christian. So I thought, well, this is going to be an interesting conversation. Of course, by then, he already had a hint of what we were about to talk about because he and I went to dinner together, just the two of us, which we had never done in our lives. I told him he was the very person who I thought would reject me. He looked me square in the eye and said,

"Jesus would not have rejected you, so why should I?"

I realized that that was a true Christian sitting across the table from me.

After all of that, I realized I had a gift in the love, affection, and support of my family. I was given the gift of having great people in my life. So I decided that was the moment I was going to make sure that not only was I not in the closet anymore, but I wanted to help those who were and didn't have the same gift that I was given. Coming out is important, regardless of what other people do or say. As an adult, you get to choose the people who are in your life. If you have the luxury of being able to have family that is blood relatives, then you're lucky. But if they are not supportive of you, then you can choose a family that is not blood-related, and that's okay. You can have the same life that I have; it just requires an extra step in doing so.

I came out on the radio right after that. After working at the bookstore, I got a job as a news writer for a morning radio show. We were doing a segment called Singled Out because Jenny McCarthy was hosting a dating show by the same name on MTV. We were going to do our own version, and I made the comment,

"Are you going to do a gay version?"

And the host said to me,

"Why, are you volunteering?"

"Well, if it gets it on the radio, then I will volunteer."

And that's how I came out. MTV had not even done a gay version yet, but I was on air getting a date with a woman. That made me the first full-time morning show personality that came out in Atlanta. I served on that show for a couple of more years. Following that, I served on a show called "The Bert Show" in Atlanta, and that really brought my name to the forefront. When Bert interviewed me for the job and asked if I had questions for him, my response was,

"I'm a lesbian, and I will not pretend I'm not. The only way I'll take the job is if I'm out on the air."

He explained he wouldn't want me to be anybody other than who I was. Bert was very supportive, as were all the members of the Bert Show on and off-air. I was on the Bert show for 10 years and talked about everything in my life. When I left the show, I took a hiatus from the morning radio. That's when Chick-fil-A was under fire for donating funds to an organization that was involved in transitional therapy, which meant they tried to make gay people straight. There were protests against that. So they did customer appreciation day to counter the protest, the idea being if you're someone who believes in the company's rights to spend their money as they wish, then come and celebrate with a discount on food. It became an anti-gay event, and there were throngs of people that showed up. Bert called me and asked if I would come on and talk about it.

I went on the radio and said I could not care less about the people who were standing in line at Chick-fil-A. I wanted the 14-year-olds, the 10-year-olds, and the 16-year-olds that were listening and watching this, who were scared, who were identifying that chicken sandwich rally as a reason to hate themselves if they were gay, or to hate their friends who were gay. I told them that all these people were on the wrong side of history, that you follow your God, and you follow your hearts. Any act of inclusion is something that's good, and any act of exclusion is something that will never last.

I later got a job at B98.5 in Atlanta, which is traditionally a very conservative radio station. They had no problem with me being out on the air, which I hope further inspired young gays and lesbians to learn to love themselves for who they are. I was also given the opportunity to be a part of a syndicated show. It was based out of New York, and they had a New York host and an LA host. They were trying to find a lesbian that wasn't some caricature, who was already in broadcasting, and they came upon me in Atlanta.

I got the job because I was the only out lesbian that wasn't a caricature in the country.

I was born the way I am, but I had to stifle my voice for so long. I had to lie, and I had to suffer. I had to mourn the loss of so many significant years of fun because being gay was not fun at all in the beginning. If there had been a radio personality talking about her life on air when I was 14, then maybe I could have had more fun. I was lucky enough to be one of the first and was successful. I think that what makes success is authenticity.

My son is being raised by two mothers. We're both confident women, but we weren't sure how to approach the topic with him. We weren't sure how to make it not weird for him. Do we tell him ahead of time that this is going to be an issue for other people? Or do we wait until other people make it an issue? One day his other mother was taking him through a grocery store when he was 2 or 3. When they were at the checkout, he looked at the cashier and announced he had two moms. "I've got two moms." The cashier responded what made him feel very lucky. We had never said a word to him, yet he already recognized that there was something different about his life. And he had the confidence to put us out as a toddler that I didn't have until I was 25-years-old.

I want to be a role model for my son so he can draw from all of my experiences and understand that whatever his life is, whatever minority situations he faces as an adult, inclusion is always the right thing to do. It's a lesson I'm still learning. Religion has been used as such a weapon against the gay community. I was raised in a church family, and I took myself out of it because I didn't want to face that. I'd heard enough about how the church felt about people like me. I have to go back to the church environment; I have to include those things in my life, and I have to walk the walk. I have to include people even though I don't agree with them. I have to include people from those walks of life who were raised that I was wrong. It's okay for us to be different.

The way you learn about yourself in the world around you is by opening yourself up to the things that are different from you. I think the sooner we get to where difference is not a threat, the better. So in my little lesbian world, if I can help women and men feel better about themselves for being gay, or if I can just help people feel better about themselves, then it's all worth it. There's an entire population of people who go to bed lonely because they feel alone. They feel that nobody sees them or understands them, or worst of all, that they're not lovable. I'm the small-town girl who started out saying, *Oh, God, I'm gay.* I'm evolving into the woman that says, *Thank God, I'm gay.* And that's how I'll live the rest of my life.

Melissa Carter

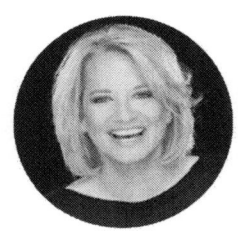

Children's Author, Radio and Podcast Personality

Melissa Carter is a familiar voice in Atlanta, having served as a member of morning shows on 99X, Q100 and B8.5. She was also part of a nationally-syndicated team on the Westwood One radio network, and has been honored with several awards for her work. A public speaker, columnist, and children's book author Melissa currently hosts her podcast, "The Friendzy," that is dedicated to empowering women over 40. It can be heard weekly anywhere you listen to podcasts and seen on The Friendzy's Youtube channel.

https://www.glaad.org/resourcelist
https://pflag.org/hotlines

The Black Card

I was born in the late 1970s as the middle child of four children. Being the middle child created many insecurities. I later knew I was experiencing something called "Middle Child Syndrome." Middle Child Syndrome is where you are unseen, overlooked, and you're not really heard. And because of this, I always felt like the black sheep of the family.

When I was nine, my mom and dad divorced, creating a really difficult time for all of us. And my mom was left to raise four girls. Because of this, her love was a tough love. Today I understand, as it must have been difficult being a single black female raising four girls alone.

As a child, I had dreams. One of which was to be a dental hygienist. Never had I dreamed it would be the place that I would really see the magnitude of racism and how big of an impact it had on my life. It started while I was part of a work-study program at my college.

It was during this works-study program that I had the moment that opened my eyes to hardcore racism. I happened to overhear a conversation between two women in the office. One of them stated that because of affirmative action, the college had to make sure that they admitted at least a few "black" students into the hygiene program. I was baffled. Why just a few?? Why only 2%?

Now I knew this was the reason why I was selected for this specific program. I became one of those "two percenters" in the program. The school made it hard for us. They often singled us out in our academics. They even held one of the ladies back because they felt that she wasn't "good enough."

Despite this, I pushed on, and I graduated! This was one of the best moments of my life. Entering the dental hygiene world, I realized that out of all employed dental hygienists, 2% of them are black women. 2%? Inequality and racism exist everywhere.

I continued to excel as a dental hygienist. However, in my heart, I knew I wanted to be a mother. Years later, after overcoming a 12-year battle of infertility, I became pregnant. After delivering our daughter, my husband and I agreed that I would become a full-time mom. So,

I quit my full-time job as a dental hygienist and became a full-time mom and entrepreneur.

I was excited about this new chapter in my life, but there was a problem. Entering the entrepreneur world made me feel small. How? Why? My business is direct sales. And in this business, there were not a lot of women who looked like me. There were a lot of women who were white women, and they were all top earners.

I looked at those women like, *this is impossible for me, I could never earn more than I felt that I could earn in business.* I found myself, again, battling the Middle Child Syndrome. I had a ton of limiting beliefs. Well, I proved myself wrong. I became a top seller within the first six months of business. I was ecstatic!!

Yet, it felt weird. I felt alone and out of place. I felt their energy; I felt as if no one wanted me around. The white women I worked with made me feel like an outcast. One even went as far as to say to call me Bozo The Clown because of my red dreadlocks. I am not making this up! It is true! She felt that I should dye my hair a more natural color since I was a top earner.

Eventually, I decided it was time for me to leave. I started building my personal brand, showing people who I wanted them to believe I was. I now know I was calling myself a Shot Caller when I really wasn't a Shot Caller! I was still this unseen individual in the world. I knew I had these talents of deep insight when it comes to business because I am a lifelong learner (I have always consumed books since I was a little girl). I knew I had these gifts that I needed to share with the world. But how do I get them out there? How do I connect with the right people?

I tried many times to pitch my service to women that were white, and no one wanted it. The truth is, I've always felt inferior to white women in this industry. That's the norm. It's the culture where white women are seen as being better than black women; they are presumed to be more intelligent than us and that they know more than us.

Being born in this world as a black person is strike one, but being black and a female entrepreneur can be disenfranchising. As black female entrepreneurs, we must work harder and lower our rates, which in turn decreases our confidence and sense of self-worth. Yes, this has slowly been changing since 2020, but there are still so many hurdles to still overcome.

I knew I had it in me, but what helped me to realize that I knew my shit was when I was asked to create a strategic plan for a startup company. The lady (black) messaged me on Facebook, and she asked me for my help. I was all in! I worked with her for six months. Her direct sales company, which she started from the ground up, now currently has 400 members because of working with me.

This win truly affirmed my brilliance to myself but made me wonder why is it only my "kind" who invests in me and hires me? Honestly, most black entrepreneurs are much quicker to invest in white coaches than blacks. Why? Stereotypes are why! Because we grew up with the false image that white people were superior to us, and because they attended the better schools, they were smarter than us.

I must confess that even to this day, I feel uncomfortable pitching white women my service. Why? Because I was denied so many times. I felt like I couldn't be in that circle. I felt weird being in that space.

However, I am changing. I'm finding the more I love who I am, the more I believe in what I know and what I offer. All people need me, they need my voice, they need my brilliance, and they need my story.

If we are all honest, we all need each other. Right? We all live together on planet Earth. We all bleed red.

I must state that I do not think that all white people are racist, but there are many who are. Some are not publicly displaying it, but they do it privately. However, it is easy to see if you are a spiritually aligned individual. There is a certain presence or aura that you can feel when you are around a person that is trying to hide it. There may even be some reading this chapter and thinking, "Here we go again!" Here is the deal, we will continue to see these issues happen if it is not viewed from an intersectional perspective.

Black people believe we all need each other and are not racist. If we see ANYONE that we can benefit from learning from, we invest our money and time, no matter the color. If we see that it will benefit our well-being, we invest. And in return, we contribute a trillion dollars a year into this economy and are least likely to receive access to funding when we start our own business or just to invest in our business growth.

We need to stretch ourselves and continue to learn. So, I joined a high-level coaching group where there were only three black women, and guess what? The coach is a white female. Now, I have known this woman for many years, and she has always "seen" me. She has invited me on her stages to speak, and she has called me out when she knows that I am playing down my greatness, and she makes me feel comfortable in her space. When I told one of my business besties (a black female) that I was investing in this high-level program, she said, "Represent us! You got this! Show them who we are!" And I said, "I must!"

I know I am speaking about something not many black women speak about. Writing this makes me super uncomfortable because inequality and racism in business is an uncomfortable subject. But I must speak. I hope that my story galvanizes the entrepreneurship world and ignites other black female entrepreneurs to start speaking their truth.

We have to start talking about how structural racism exists not only in corporations but in the entrepreneurial sector. For instance, did you know that it takes black women 20 months to get paid for what a white man gets paid in 12 months? This shit is happening to so many of us, but we are not talking about it. We store a lot of pain when it comes to our experiences with racism, and that burden gets heavy.

When it comes to entrepreneurship, this is a huge dragon that most black women and men deal with, and I have been wanting to speak about it for years but have refrained. Why do black female entrepreneurs never talk about this? One word...Fear! Fear of losing relationships with our white counterparts. Fear of exposure. Fear of being targeted. Fear of rejection.

The good news is black female entrepreneurs are breaking through glass ceilings. We own HALF of all female-owned companies in the United States. Rhianna, the famous singer, just recently shattered the glass ceiling and became a Billionaire in the beauty industry.

However, I still see that we, as black women, feel like we need to do everything in our business and not ask for help. Note to my sisters: *You do not need to be all things in your business; it is ok for you to delegate in your business and meditate daily in order to stay aligned with your truest self and focus on your core competencies.* I can tell you this as a black female, we often shy away from asking for the help we need because society labels us as "Strong black women." Well, it is time to pivot from this way of thinking because being strong can keep you broke!

As a black female entrepreneur, I can say that our dragon is not always about racism, but it is also how we treat each other. A mental block that we often come across is being afraid to collaborate with one another because one of the belief that one may become better than the other. Collaborations are designed to give all parties involved more exposure. Just this statement alone should change the narrative on how black women approach collaborating in business. Note to my sisters: *when we see each other moving up levels in this entrepreneurship game, clap for one another, empower each other, let's look each other in the eye and say, "well done." Bitterness doesn't get you far; it only keeps you in a stuck place. Let us edify one another and understand that our journeys to this road to riches are different, but we can land at the same destination.*

Overall, I truly hope that this entire story changes the narrative on how black female and male entrepreneurs are treated in the business sector. I must constantly remind myself that things are always working out for me. Writing this story, I know that my story needs to be heard. I am in faith that I am in the right place at the right time.

And when I feel self-doubt or imposter syndrome trying to settle in, I remind myself that we are all seeking the highest truest self as human beings. The only difference is our talents and the way we choose to show up in this world.

I remind myself that I am beautiful. I remind myself that I am brilliant. I remind myself that there are people waiting for me to show up. I remind myself to be the best version of Tequila Cousar.

I would like to end with this, *"What does it serve to not have this conversation?"*

Tequila Cousar

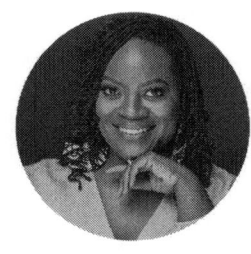

Personal Branding Coach

Tequila Cousar is a well-respected Speaker,Personal Branding Coach, and #1 International Best Selling Author in Columbus, Ohio. She has over a decade of entrepreneurial insight and expertise. She helps Lady Bosses build their online persona and monetize their purpose.

www.tequilacousar.com

https://thewomenscenter.org/black-mental-health-resources/

https://www.vogue.com/article/black-womens-health-support-organizations

Acknowledgements

This book has been a huge passion project for me. It is because of all of the women who have shared their stories through tears, hugs and laughs that I was called to collect the women on these pages to share *their* stories of triumph over tragedy. There are some women who come immediately to mind when I think of all of the women I have met over the years, that were a part of the inspiration for this project. (there are so many I could never list you all)

My mother, Norma Mansfield-McDonough, the first surthrivor I ever met in life. Aurea McGarry, who catapulted my speaking authority on her Live Your Legacy Summit stage and then taking me under her wing to show me how to make bigger, better impact. Jennifer Riis-Poulsen, who has dedicated her business to helping women Power Up through self defense empowerment both physically and mentally. Jada Boisvert and Shannon Wilson, for being two of the original Super Women when I started my own events, that showed me how much impact women can have on each other. Doree O'Neal and Carla-Jayne Hollingworth for becoming instant Star sisters and helping me navigate a few dragons along the way this year. Most of all, my best friend Nola Comingore, for always, ALWAYS loving me through every version of myself. Good, bad, emotionally illogical and empowering...sometimes all in one day.

Tell Your Story!

Do you have a story you know can impact another woman? Are you ready to make a difference and be seen and heard? Reach out to Melissa to find out how you can tell your story in a powerful way and become a best selling author.

Contact her through her website at TheLipstickCEO.com/tell-my-story

Made in the USA
Middletown, DE
08 November 2021

51479100R00119